# Workplace Skills and Professional Issues in Speech-Language Pathology

# Workplace Skills and Professional Issues in Speech-Language Pathology

**Betsy Partin Vinson**

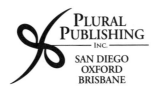

PLURAL
PUBLISHING
INC.

SAN DIEGO
OXFORD
BRISBANE

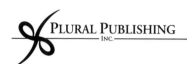

PLURAL PUBLISHING
INC.

5521 Ruffin Road
San Diego, CA 92123

e-mail: info@pluralpublishing.com
Web site: http://www.pluralpublishing.com

49 Bath Street
Abingdon, Oxfordshire OX14 1EA
United Kingdom

**FSC**
**Mixed Sources**
Product group from well-managed
forests and other controlled sources

Cert no. SW-COC-002283
www.fsc.org
© 1996 Forest Stewardship Council

Library of Congress Cataloging-in-Publication Data

Vinson, Betsy Partin.
  Workplace skills and professional issues in speech-language pathology/ Betsy Vinson.
       p. ; cm.
  Includes bibliographical references and index.
  ISBN-13: 978-1-59756-203-4 (alk. paper)
  ISBN-10: 1-59756-203-3 (alk. paper)
  1.  Speech therapy—Practice. 2.  Speech therapists—Professional ethics.  I. Title.
  [DNLM: 1.  Speech-Language Pathology. 2.  Ethics, Professional. 3.  Legislation,
Medical. 4.  Practice Management, Medical. 5.  Professional Competence.
WL 340.2 V788w 2008]
  RC428.5.V56 2008
  616.85'50068—dc22

                                                                    2008038402

# Contents

# Preface

*Workplace Skills and Professional Issues in Speech-Language Pathology* is, admittedly, a bit of a hodge-podge approach to knowledge needed to succeed in the workplace that oftentimes does not get covered in our curriculum. With the expanding Scope of Practice in our field, and the emphasis on the acquisition of specific knowledge and skills, there is little to no time to address issues such as, "What do I do if I disagree with one of my colleagues?" or "What does the law say about inclusion?" It is those types of questions, which largely have come from my students, that led to my attempts to teach these topics in our weekly "clinicians' meetings." I have also heard back from former students saying this knowledge has been useful to them in their professional settings. These letters confirmed that I should put some of this down in print to share with other individuals. The book is geared toward new professionals, but also can be used to teach graduate students about the issues they will face when they enter the work force.

As part of my preparation for the writing of this book, I compiled a survey that was disbursed to practicum supervisors asking them a variety of questions such as, "What is your best organizational strategy?" and "On a scale of 0 to 5, with 0 being the lowest, how would you rank the stress level of your job?" The findings of this survey are found in Chapters 13 and 17. I would like to extend my thanks to my fellow supervisors and friends in the Southeast University Clinical Educators (SEUCE) for helping me disseminate the questionnaire, and also to those who took the time to complete the study and return it to me. The amount of interest shown in this survey further confirmed for me that this book needed to be written.

I would also like to extend my thanks to my family for their interest in this project and their support throughout the writing. My husband, Tim, helped to keep supper on the table and dirty dishes in the dishwasher, and my children all called periodically to inquire about the progress (I'm an empty nester—maybe I should write a chapter on the joys and stresses of being an empty nester!). Finally, I would like to thank the staff at Plural Publishing for their support, encouragement, and assistance in this project.

It is my sincere wish that you, the reader, find this information useful as you go through your career.

*This book is respectfully dedicated to the students with whom I have had the privilege and pleasure of interacting as a thanks for all they have taught me.*

# SECTION I

## Getting the Job

# Chapter 1

# Resume Preparation and Interviewing

## Introduction

In today's fast-paced world, it is not uncommon for an individual to have more than two different jobs or careers over the span of their postgraduate years. Thus, a discussion of how to write a resume, the different types of resumes, and interviewing skills seemed like an appropriate way to begin a book on workplace skills.

According to the Bureau of Labor Statistics (BLS), baby boomers (born between the years 1957–1984) have held an average of 9.6 jobs between the ages of 18 to 36. They defined a job as any uninterrupted period of work with a designated employer. Men typically held 9.9 jobs, and women held 9.3 jobs. The BLS does not have data on the number of career changes over a typical American's life span. Although the Department of Labor does not keep statistics on the number of career changes due to difficulty in defining a career change, there are ballpark estimates that Americans change careers three to seven times over the span of their working years after schooling has ended.

## Resume Preparation

One's resume is often the first impression a potential employer may have of the job seeker. Thus, providing information on how to write an effective resume is the goal of this chapter. When preparing a resume, remember that the primary purpose of your resume is to market yourself and convince employers to interview you.

Most resumes are scanned in 20 seconds. To make yours stand out and warrant further attention, choose a format that draws the eye toward skills that tie directly to the employer's requirements. The resume should be visually appealing. Use plenty of white space and wide margins to draw the employer's attention to your most significant qualifications. Use bullets and short, succinct paragraphs. Powerful action words that convey strength and conviction of purpose will attract the attention of the potential employer and set you apart from others against whom you are competing. Examples of such action words are "designed," "implemented," "organized," developed," "spearheaded," and so on.

Because potential employers often receive a large number of resumes, it is suggested that the resume be a maximum of 2 pages in length. Make every word count in conveying the essence of your qualifications in a succinct and appealing format. If you have a lengthy professional history and would like to reflect this in your resume, prepare two resumes: a short one to "whet the appetite" of your potential boss, and a longer one that can be provided upon request. You can make a note on the "application resume" indicating that a more comprehensive resume is available upon request. A curriculum vitae is an example of a longer resume.

## Types of Resumes

Generally speaking, there are three types of resumes: chronologic, functional, and curriculum vitae (Lubinski, 2007).

A chronologic resume is the most commonly used. In this type of resume, one should tie the job responsibilities and achievements to specific employers, job titles, and dates. Two advantages of a chronologic resume are that it demonstrates growth in the profession, and it is straightforward and easy to read. Recalling that most resumes are scanned in 20 seconds, this format is particularly effective. When writing a chronologic resume, you should list jobs in reverse chronologic order with the most recent job first. A disadvantage of this type of resume is that it clearly emphasizes job changes and shows periods of unemployment. Thus, when using a chronologic resume, be prepared to answer questions regarding the periods of unemployment. Similarly, if there have been frequent job changes, be ready to explain why you typically do not stay in a job for an extended period of time. A second disadvantage of a chronologic resume is that it dilutes the impact of skills acquired in various settings. Thus, you should prepare a brief presentation in which you can elaborate on the skills learned in previous jobs that can be applied to the job you are seeking.

A second type of resume is the functional resume. A functional resume focuses on skills that have been learned instead of where and when the skills were developed. When writing this type of resume, you should outline the functions of the type of position for which you are applying, then insert things that you have done that pertain to each area. An advantage of a functional resume is that it helps you to sell yourself based on the skills and competencies you have to offer that may not be reflected in your recent job history (or a chronologic resume). A second advantage is that it is adaptable to special circumstances, such as lack of direct experience in a chosen field, or difficult to explain job gaps or changes. There are two main disadvantages of a functional resume. One is that your employment goals must clearly reflect the objectives of the position for which you are applying (thus, your resume will need to be tailored specifically for the particular position). Secondly, a functional resume can leave the impression that you are hiding something because it does not clearly delineate your job history. Some potential employers may see the functional resume as an attempt to "gloss over" periods of unemployment, or frequent job changes that can reflect poor performance and/or lack of dedication and commitment to a company/employer (Cole & McNichol, 1997).

A curriculum vitae is used primarily in the academic world and emphasizes one's educational background and published and presented works. In a curriculum vitae, one should describe his or her accomplishments and achievements, not activities. It is best to use a variety of action words such as those listed in the section on chronologic resumes. The primary disadvantage is that these types of resumes tend to be quite lengthy. Thus, it may be a good idea to take a chronologic format for page one, then move into the listing/description of publications, presentations, and professional activities.

In summary, if you have submitted a chronologic resume, be prepared to discuss your career history (in the order on your resume) when you are being interviewed, with most of the focus being on the most recent job(s). If using a functional resume, focus on your skills and how you developed them. The curriculum vitae is a somewhat specialized vitae that is typically used in academic settings. When being interviewed by a potential employer in an academic setting, be prepared to elaborate on your publications and presentations, and to explain the nature of your research, including grant support (or lack of). The resume should "whet the appetite" of the potential employer to learn more about you and how you can "fit into" and enhance his or her company.

### *Essential Content of Resumes*

Information that should always be included is listed below:

Name, address, telephone number, and E-mail address

Employment/career objectives

Dates of your current and previous employment(s)

Name and addresses of past and current employers

Current and past job titles

Name of university you attended

Degrees and honors earned

Graduation date(s)

Accreditation and licensure information

Professional training (on-the-job)

Professional affiliations

Publications and patents

Languages spoken fluently

Relevant skills

As a rule, the following information should not be included on a resume:

Health or physical description

Race, sex, age, or national origin

Marital status or information regarding children

Religion or church affiliations

Photographs

Hobbies/avocations

Political preferences

Salary (current or desired)

References (include on a separate sheet if asked)

Written testimonials

Pronouns such as I, we, and they

However, Lubinski (2007) points out that some of these items (e.g., hobbies, church affiliation, and children) may provide some insight into you as a person, and could serve as "starters" for the interview.

## *Personalized Cover Letters*

A cover letter should be included with every resume. The purpose of the cover letter is to establish a relationship and build a bridge to meeting the potential employer in person. It should be addressed to a specific person (title and last name; e.g., Dr. Jackson); be sure you have spelled the name correctly. The letter should be tailored to the organization, and include comments about the organization to demonstrate your familiarity of the site where one is seeking employment. When possible, also comment directly about the person to whom you are writing. This can include statements such as, "I would value the opportunity to learn from an employer such as yourself who has vast experiences in this area." This also is a good opportunity to tell something about your background that relates directly to the organization's mission, objectives, and characteristics.

### Other Cover Letters

Cover letters can be written for a variety of purposes. Therefore, one should always state the reason for the letter. Name the specific position in which you are interested. Indicate how you learned about the vacant position, why you are interested in the position. In addition, demonstrate some knowledge of the organization and what you can do for the employer. An employer wants to know that you have researched his organization and have carefully considered how you can enhance the program/agenda of his site. For example, if you have expertise in the assessment of voice disorders, discuss how your knowledge and skills in this area can be used to develop/expand/enhance the current programmatic emphases as they currently exist in the facility in which you are seeking employment. Demonstrate vision without being grandiose. Another example would be to indicate how you would reach an underserved population in the geographic area served by your potential employer. Indigent adults are often an underserved group, so you may want to indicate potential funding sources that could be tapped for grants to provide speech-language assessment and treatment for these individuals.

Explain how your background makes you a qualified candidate for the position. Point out specific achievements and/or unique qualifications, without simply repeating what is on your resume. Indicate a desire to interview and flexibility with regard to the time and place. Also, indicate that you will call in about a week to follow up and be sure the resume was received (Lubinski, Golper, & Frattali, 2007).

## *References*

List the name, address, telephone number, and e-mail address of the person who is providing a reference. Include a sentence on your resume explaining your relationship with that reference. Let your references know to expect a call (from whom and when). Explain to your reference why you are seeking that specific position, and why it is a "good fit."

## The Interview: A Two-Way Fact-Finding Mission

An interview is a mutual exploration to see if there is a "fit" between you, the organization, and what the employer wants. As the interviewee, one should gain an understanding of the organization's values, culture, and business issues. For the employer, it is a chance to gain insight into whether you can make a contribution to their organization and fit into their culture.

Of course, a critical item in this fact-finding mission is to inquire about the salary. The individual should provide a range and be willing to accept the low end of the range. However, the salary is not the only consideration. It is important to take into consideration the entire compensation package, including benefits, because sometimes a lower salary may be offset by more benefits. It is reasonable to request the following items as benefits: dues for memberships in profession organizations (i.e., ASHA, state associations, special interest divisions, etc.), vacation, sick leave, professional leave, retirement and investment considerations, and insurance (health, life, dental, long-term care). You should also compare factors specific to the geographic areas where you are seeking employment. This would include the average cost of utilities, access to medical care, average cost of housing, availability of a variety of community services, driving distance to work, efficiency of public transportation, income tax (state and local), cost of living index, availability of public recreation, area crime rate, and the like. If you have children, how does the school system compare to those in other areas where you are seeking employment? Are there after-school programs available and if so, what is the average cost of child care?

## *Preparing for the Interview*

The day before your interview, drive the route at the same time of day as your interview so you can estimate how long the drive will take. Plan to arrive 10 to 15 minutes before your interview. Pay particular attention to your appearance. Wear professional attire, and be well-groomed. Do not wear excessive jewelry, and suits typically are appropriate for men and women (be sure they fit well). Clothing should be understated but professional.

Second, learn as much as you can about the organization prior to the interview. Find out how many employees they have, the mission and vision of the organization, the presence of the organization in the local community, and the general structure of the organization.

Finally, if possible, explore the needs of the organization. Do they have a niche into which you can bring your expertise to help them broaden the services they provide? For example, if applying to a school district, having expertise in reading and spelling disorders may be a part of the job that has not been addressed in the past. If applying to a hospital, does the potential employer have areas of need such as someone with expertise in, for example, dysphagia or treatment for laryngectomees? If so, what knowledge and experience do you have that would help your potential employer fill these needs in his or her program (Cole & McNichol, 1997)?

## *In the Interview*

I would like to point out that one should treat the support staff with respect and courtesy. Usually, a job applicant will check in with the potential employer's secretary/administrative assistant. Treat the outer office staff the same way you would treat your interviewer. This individual is very likely to report to the employer on your demeanor and interaction with the staff, as well as how you conducted yourself while waiting to be interviewed.

One of the most critical elements in the interview is to demonstrate that you are a team player. If you have had a previous job, discuss how you fit into that organization, and what your role(s) was(were) in your previous position. Be inquisitive, inquiring how the employer sees you fitting into his or her organization. Listen carefully and think before you speak. Do not feel pressured to fill a moment of silence. Pause briefly to think about a question, but do not fill the space with "uhs," "ums," and "you know."

Smile frequently and inject some enthusiasm into your voice. Restrict questions to those concerning the job and its duties. Never criticize a former employer, your professors, or anyone with whom you have been associated.

### Handling Questions

Answering questions from the potential employer is an opportunity to show your personality and willingness to assume the roles that the employer envisions. Many of these questions could create a lengthy response. Thus, you should carefully review these questions and practice responses that do not exceed two minutes in length. Some of the questions the employer may ask include the following (*Note:* The following sets of questions are compiled from lists developed by Cole & McNichol, 1997, and by Lubinski, Golper, & Frattali, 2007):

1. Why did you choose the profession?
2. What are your ambitions or long-range goals and how might this job help you reach them?
3. What have you done that you are particularly proud of?
4. Have you ever refused a job or promotion? If yes, describe the situation.
5. Tell me about a responsibility you enjoyed. What did you do to meet that responsibility?
6. What do you consider your greatest strengths and weaknesses?
7. What are your specific interests within the field?
8. What two or three accomplishments have given you the most satisfaction? Why? (Cole & McNichol, 1997; Lubinski, 2007; Rasberry & Lindsay, 1994)

The interviewer will, most likely, inquire about your academic background. Be prepared to discuss the clinical education you participated in, including a list of your practica/externships. He or she also may ask, "What professional conferences/workshops have you attended?" Rarely has the author heard of a potential employer requesting a transcript showing the applicant's grades, but the employer may ask what college classes you liked the least or most, and why.

The interviewer will want to evaluate your skills in communication. An interviewer may ask the interviewee to tell him or her about a time when he or she had a project that required interacting with people at different levels within an organization. How did you do this? What caused you the most problems in executing your tasks? With whom were you most comfortable/uncomfortable and why? The employer may also ask if the interviewee would feel comfortable delivering a presentation to the professionals in the structure of the facility.

The potential employer will also want to address the following questions to see how prepared the interviewee is with regard to knowing the company. Some of these include:

1. Why are you seeking a job with us?
2. What do you know about our organization? How did you learn that?
3. What would you expect out of this job?
4. What do you like best about this job? What do you like the least?

14. What would be a reason that you would not treat a person? (Cole & McNichol, 1997; Lubinski, 2007; Rasberry & Lindsay, 1994)

**Energy and Organization.** Employers are always seeking to find high-energy employees who can carry their loads without becoming too stressed and, thereby begin to be unhappy and unsatisfactory employees. This issue is dealt with in Chapter 17, "Stress and Burnout." Typically, there are three questions related to energy and organization to expect from an interviewer:

1. How large a caseload could you handle?
2. What challenges do you normally face in getting things done?
3. Describe a project that required a high amount of energy over a long period of time. What did you do to keep your enthusiasm up? When you have a great deal of work to do that requires extra time and effort, where does your energy come from?

**Getting Along with People.** Employers want to hire individuals with good "people skills." To that end, the interviewee should be prepared to answer the following questions:

1. Tell me about a time when you needed to get an understanding of another person's situation before you could get your job done. How did you gain their understanding, and what problems did you encounter?
2. What is your role as a group member? Tell me about a specific accomplishment you achieved as a group member and what your role was.
3. Describe some of the different styles of people you have worked with in the past and what kind of approaches you took to work effectively with them.
4. How would you define a cooperative environment?
5. Tell me about when a team fell apart. Why did it happen? What did you do?
6. Have you ever had to build motivation or team spirit with coworkers? Tell me about the situation.
7. How would you handle a patient who broke down and cried?
8. What experience do you have with managing conflicts?
9. How do you handle criticism? (Cole & McNichol, 1997; Lubinski, 2007; Rasberry & Lindsay, 1994)

**Motivation.** Questions about the interviewee's motivation can provide insights into his or her driving force and what he or she finds to be reinforcing. Specifically, an interviewer may ask the following questions:

1. What can you do for us that someone else cannot do?
2. Tell me about a time when you felt that your contributions had been appropriately recognized.
3. What kinds of rewards are most satisfying to you?
4. How does this affect what you do in your job? How does this affect the effort you put into your job?
5. For what are you most frequently criticized, and by whom? (Cole & McNichol, 1997; Lubinski, 2007; Rasberry & Lindsay, 1994)

### Responding to Inappropriate Interview Questions

Occasionally an interviewer will ask an inappropriate question. Typically, these questions center around national origin, age and/or gender, health, physical information, and marital and/or family status. Examples of these inappropriate questions and an acceptable answer are given below:

National Origin

*Questions:* Are you a U.S. citizen? Where were you born? What is your native language?

*Answer:* I am legally eligible to work in the United States. I speak both Spanish and English fluently.

Age

*Question:* How old are you? Please state your date of birth.

*Answer:* I am over the age of 18 and eligible for work.

Marital/Family Status

*Questions:* What is your marital status? How many children do you have? Do you plan on starting a family soon? Describe your child care arrangements.

*Answer:* I can meet the work schedule that this position requires.

Golper, & Frattali, 2007). If interviewed by a team, send a note to each member of the team. In this note, the interviewee can offer clarification of any responses that, upon reflection, you did not answer well. Furthermore, this is an opportunity to add any relevant information you omitted from the interview. Finally, one should call attention to the most important aspects of the position and express your confidence in your ability to handle it.

## Summary

Typically, one sends a resume with a cover letter and receives a letter or telephone call from the future employer to come in for an interview. Rework your resume into a 2-minute verbal introduction. Use this 2-minute introduction when you are networking and to respond to the interview statement, "Tell me about yourself." Write out the introduction and practice it in front of a mirror with a tape or digital recorder.

Remember, when networking, provide a 30-second summary of your career. State the type of work you have been doing and a description of the setting. Use one sentence to explain why you are looking for a job. Then, mention the setting and position you are hoping to get. Ask a question that will encourage two-way conversations. In interviewing, your introduction should include a statement of why the person should hire you. Make this sentence one that you would like the employer to repeat when describing your attributes. Dedicate your statements to the position and setting at hand.

Following the introduction, ask the employer if he or she has any points on which he or she would like for you to elaborate. An interview can be somewhat stressing, so one should adopt body language that conveys comfort with the interviewer and confidence that you are the right person for the job opening. In addition, employers will be impressed with your knowledge of the facility because this indicates the interviewee's ability to gather pertinent information on which to base his or her questions. Just as important as the interview are your actions following the interview. Writing a thank-you note to everyone involved in your interview is a way to make a final good impression on the employer.

# References

Cole, P. A., & McNichol, J. G. (1997). *Tools for a successful job search.* Rockville, MD: ASHA.

Lubinski, R. (2007). Preparing for employment. In R. Lubinski, L. C. Golper, & C. M. Frattali (Eds.), *Professional issues in speech-language pathology and audiology* (3rd ed.). Clifton Park, NY: Thomson Delmar Learning.

Rasberry, R. W., & Lindsay, L. L. (1994). *Effective managerial communication.* Belmont, CA: Wadsworth.

# SECTION II

# Things You
# Should Know

# Chapter 2

# Information to Know

## (WHO, Health Care Reform, ASHA Documents, Workplace Settings, Malpractice and Liability)

## Introduction

According to the World Health Organization, approximately 600 million individuals across the globe live with various types of disabilities, many of them due to fallout from living in impoverished conditions as well as disabilities due to "chronic diseases, injuries, violence, infectious diseases, and malnutrition." (WHO Web site, retrieved 3/28/08). Thus, there are many issues with which the speech-language pathologist must deal during the course of a professional lifetime. The purpose of this chapter is to provide an overview of some of these issues, definitions, and practices for the purpose of having an easy reference.

### *Definitions of Impairment, Disability, and Handicap as They Relate to Communication Disorders*

The World Health Organization (WHO) is an agency of the United Nations that serves as a coordinator on globally identified issues related to public health. It was established on April 7, 1948 and is headquartered in Geneva, Switzerland. WHO "is responsible for providing leadership on global health matters, shaping the health research agenda, setting norms and standards, articulating evidence-based policy options, providing technical support to countries and monitoring and assessing health trends" (WHO Web site, retrieved 3/28/08).

The World Health Organization's (WHO) International Classification of Impairments, Disabilities, and Handicaps (ICIDH), currently has two classifications in development. The ICIDH initially was based on a biomedical model that targeted causes and cures, but, over time, has become an integrated biopsychological model of disablement and human functioning. Through this model, the ICIDH has expanded its perspective to include removal of barriers that interfere with routine daily activities and quality of life issues (Frattali, 1999).

WHO defines "disabilities as an umbrella term, covering impairments, activity limitations, and participation restrictions. An impairment is a problem in body function or structure; an activity limitation is a difficulty encountered by an individual in executing a task or action; while participation is a problem experienced by an individual in involvement in life situations. Thus, disability is a complex phenomenon, reflecting an interaction between features of a person's body and features of the society in which he or she lives" (WHO Web site, 2008).

Frattali (1999) adapted the definitions of impairment, disability, and handicap and applied them to speech-language pathology as follows:

*Impairment:* "specific speech, language, swallowing, or cognitive deficits" (Frattali, 1999, p. 32), (i.e., patient has slow transit of food through pharyngeal and esophageal stages);

*Disability:* "the effects of the impairment(s) on everyday communication or eating activities" (Frattali, 1999, p. 32), (i.e., patient has to eat a modified diet);

*Handicap:* "a range of social effects as defined by the work place or school system, family, relationships, community roles, etc." (Frattali, 1999, p. 32.), (i.e., patient eats alone).

The ICIDH was created in 1980 by WHO "to provide a unifying framework for classifying the consequences of disorder" (http://www.cdc.gov/nchs, 2008). Since 1993, the WHO Collaborating Center for the Family of International Classifications for North America (housed in the National Center for Health Statistics; formerly the North America Collaborating Center—NACC), has coordinated revisions of the ICIDH. On May 22, 2001, the ICIDH was revised and approved under a new name, the International Classification of Functioning, Disability, and Health (ICF). The ICF has 3 components: (1) Body functions and structure; (2) Activities (individual's tasks and actions) and participation (involvement in life events); and (3) Additional information on severity and environmental factors.

A modification of the original ICIDH codes has been made to reflect a new social understanding of disability and describe the dimensions of functioning and disablement at three levels: the body, the person, and society. Definitions of these levels of functioning are:

*Impairment*: a loss or abnormality of body structure or of a physiologic or psychological function (e.g., loss of speech, loss of vision);

*Activity*: the nature and extent of functioning at the level of the person (i.e., taking care of oneself, communication activities, activities required of a job); activities may be limited in nature, duration, and quality;

*Participation*: the nature and extent of a person's involvement in life situations in relation to impairment, activities, health conditions, and contextual factors (i.e., being employed, participating in community events, ability to do both). Participation may be restricted in nature, duration, and quality (Frattali, 1999, p. 32).

Disabilities, regardless of whether they are chronic or sudden in nature, typically have a negative impact on body image, self-concept, ego, and identity. Therefore, when determining the impact of disability, it is important to understand patient and family dynamics and their emotional states because it may affect how one interprets the progress of the patient during and after rehabilitation (Dikengil, 1998).

The WHO adopted a resolution at the 58th World Health Assembly that was focused on improving the daily lives of individuals who have disabilities, with efforts being initiated to facilitate equal opportunities for individuals with disabilities, and to uphold their "rights and dignity." Specifically, the resolution states the following:

- Promoting early intervention and identification of disability, especially for children

▧ Supporting the integration of community-based rehabilitation services into the health system

▧ Facilitating development and access to appropriate assistive devices, including wheelchairs, hearing aids, orthoses, prostheses, and so forth, which help to ensure the inclusion and participation of people with disabilities in their societies

▧ Strengthening collaborative work on disability across the United Nations system and with member states, academia, private sector and nongovernmental organizations, including disabled people's organizations

▧ Production and dissemination of a *World Report on Disability and Rehabilitation* based on the best available scientific evidence (WHO Web site, retrieved 3/28/08).

The International Classification of Functioning, Disability, and Health (abbreviated "ICF") is structured around three primary and broadly defined components:

▧ Body functions and structure

▧ Activities (related to tasks and actions by an individual) and participation (involvement in a life situation)

▧ Additional information on severity and environmental factors (http://www.cdc.gov retrieved 3/28/08).

With regard to ICF, the following is written on the Web site for the Centers for Disease Control:

Functioning and disability are viewed as a complex interaction between the health condition of the individual and the contextual factors of the environment as well as personal factors. The picture produced by this combination of factors and dimensions is of "the person in his or her world." The classification treats these dimensions as interactive and dynamic rather than linear or static. It allows for an assessment of the degree of disability, although it is not a measurement instrument. It is applicable to all people, whatever their health condition. The language of the ICF is neutral as to etiology, placing the emphasis on function rather than condition or disease. It also is carefully designed to be relevant across cultures as well as age groups and genders, making it highly appropriate for heterogeneous populations (http://www.cdc.gov, retrieved 3/28/08).

## Definitions Related to ASHA

The following definitions refer to statements issued by the American Speech-Language-Hearing Association (ASHA) (ASHA Web site, retrieved 3/28/08).

- **Scope of practice statement:** A list of professional activities that define the range of services offered within the profession of speech-language pathology.
- **Preferred practice patterns:** Statements that define generally applicable characteristics of activities directed toward individual patients/clients that address structural requisites of the practice, processes to be carried out, and expected outcomes.
- **Position statements:** Statements that specify ASHA's policy and stance on a matter that is important not only to the membership but also to other outside agencies or groups.
- **Practice guidelines:** A recommended set of procedures for a specific area of practice, based on research findings and current practice. These procedures detail the knowledge, skills, and/or competencies needed to perform the procedures effectively.

Preferred practice patterns are designated by ASHA as being "generic and universally applicable practice patterns" (ASHA, 2004), and are consistent with the designations of "functioning," "disability," and "health" as defined by the World Health Organization in their International Classification of Functioning, Disability and Health (WHO, 2001) and ASHA's Scope of Practice for Speech-Language Pathology (ASHA, 2001).

## Health Care Reform

According to Griffin and Fazen (1993), managed care:

> . . . is a system that integrates the financing and delivery of appropriate health care services. Managed care programs have certain common elements: First of all, arrangements are made with selected providers to furnish comprehensive health care providers to covered persons. In some programs, this limits the choice of providers to whom the patient

can go for services. Secondly, fees and rates which are lower than the normal price of services are negotiated with the selected providers. On most bills, there is an "amount charged" and the prenegotiated "amount allowed" column. Thirdly, formal programs exist for ongoing quality improvement and utilization review. A fourth characteristic is that significant financial incentives are offered for covered persons to use providers and procedures covered by the managed care plan. (p. 1)

There are five types of managed care organizations (MCOs):

1. Managed indemnity insurance plans: Also known as fee-for-service, participants in this type of MCO pay a monthly premium, and are reimbursed based on the billed charges. Participants may choose any licensed provider, "although the plans specify the services and types of providers that are covered" (Griffin & Fazen, 1993, p. 2).
2. Preferred provider organizations (PPOs): In PPOs, the provider or insurer negotiates a lower rate with a network of selected groups of providers. Enrollees can opt to go to a nonpreferred provider, although they will pay a higher fee, and may be limited in the service options.
3. Health maintenance organizations (HMOs): "HMOs provide a defined, comprehensive set of health services to a voluntarily enrolled population within a specified geographic services area" (Griffin & Fazen, 1993, p. 2). Members are required to seek services within the provider network. The providers are reimbursed based on a capitated amount that is pre-negotiated. There are four main types of HMOs:
   a. Staff model HMO: The HMO owns a central facility (or facilities), and the health care providers are all salaried employees.
   b. Group model: The HMO contracts with multispecialty physician group practices to provide care either in a company-owned facility or in their own offices (ASHA, 1993).
   c. Independent practice associations (IPAs): In IPAs, the physicians see the patients in their own offices, and are reimbursed under a variety of plans. The patient sees a health practitioner who has a contract with the HMO to provide services.
   d. Network: Designed to serve a large population of HMO members, the network consists of a contract between the HMO and both multispecialty groups and independent practitioners in a large geographic area (ASHA, 1993).

4. Point of service plan (POS): This is also known as the open-ended HMO. Members have the option of seeing providers who are not in the plan. However, "there is a strong financial incentive to use the affiliated providers" (Griffin & Fazen, 1993, p. 2).
5. Physician hospital organization (PHO): The PHO contracts with the MCOs to provide physician and hospital services to enrollees. All decisions are made within the network, so there is no third-party. The PHO is organized by the physician's community and hospital.

Carol Frattali (1999) outlined six influences that are currently and presently shaping "a consumer-directed approach to care": The first influence is a social definition of quality care. Excessive care is expensive and unethical. In today's health care climate, providing excessive care to one patient may, in the long run, be denying care to another patient. One must think of the impact of one's service delivery system not only on current patients, but on future patients as well.

Second, there is increased specialization in health care. As clinical and scientific knowledge expands, there is a tendency to define increased specialization which, over time, leads to fragmentation of health care. Third-party providers see increased specialization as more expensive; thus, the patient suffers because benefits for specialized tests and care are denied.

Regulatory reforms constitute a third influence. The use of clinical competence standards instead of credentials has led to dramatic changes in staffing patterns based on regulation agencies' standards. Clinicians must "both define and document their competencies to accreditation agencies and payers" (Frattali, 1998, p. 243). Those who do not do this are subject to having their competencies defined by the medical staff and/or outside agencies for which they work.

Lack of convincing treatment data is a fourth influence. Much has been said in recent years about the need for valid and reliable outcomes data that can document the effectiveness of treatment methodology employed by speech-language pathologists. It is critical that we prove that lower cost treatment alternatives result in less satisfactory outcomes both clinically and economically.

Emerging models of care are another characteristic of the consumer-driven approach to health care. "New models based on an integration of social science (e.g., the patient's perception of health, functional status, quality of life) rather than medical science paradigms (diagnosis and cure) are just recently gaining the attention of the health care community and are predicted to influence approaches to service delivery" (Frattali, 1998, p. 243). The emphasis is predicted to continue a shift toward functional outcomes, for example, dealing with useful communication tools instead of underlying language processes.

Finally, consumer choice and satisfaction drive the current health care system. Consumers have more options than ever with regard to selecting a health care plan. Thus, if they are not satisfied, they can elect to change to a different carrier. Even though many of the changes are the result of federal mandates, the market is consumer driven.

## *Managed Care Plans*

Managed care plans may be variously referred to as health maintenance organizations (HMOs), preferred provider organizations (PPOs), and independent practice associations (IPAs).

> The most sweeping changes in health care involve managed care in all its hybrid forms. Generally, managed care describes a cost-effective system that integrates both the financing and delivery of health care services. It is defined by the American Association of Health Plans (American Managed Care and Review Association, 1995), the national trade association representing managed care organizations, as a comprehensive approach to health care delivery that encompasses planning and coordination of care, patient and provider education, monitoring of care quality, and cost control. (Frattali, 1998, p. 244)

Henri and Hallowell (1999) state that there are three goals of managed care. The first is to ensure the quality and coordination of care, and the second is to create access to medical care for people who need it. However, with time, goals one and two have fallen by the wayside in favor of the third goal which is cost control. The impacts of HMOs and MCOs is felt in fee-for-service medicine as well as Medicaid and Medicare. Henri and Hallowell (1999) state the situation as follows:

> These mechanisms include increasingly stringent utilization review; pre-admission certification for hospital stays; required preauthorization for services; negotiated reduced reimbursement rates; designation of a restricted list of preferred providers; the designation of physicians as "gatekeepers" of patients' access to health care services; salaried employ-

ment of physicians by payer organizations; incentives for physicians not to refer patients to specialty services (such as rehabilitation services); use of red-flag diagnostic or treatment categories to deny reimbursement; and restrictions on frequency, intensity, and duration of care. (p. 4)

One of the primary features of managed care is the use of a "gatekeeper" who coordinates a patient's care. The gatekeeper typically is the primary care physician who must make the decisions regarding the scope and intensity of managed care. For example, a patient who is seeking speech-language therapy services would need to make the request through his or her primary care physician who then, if deemed appropriate, refers the patient for therapy (Frattali, 1999).

A second feature is utilization review (UR) which refers to the monitoring of a patient's use of health care services and resources. This would include "second opinions, precertifications, treatment authorizations, discharge planning, and chart reviews" (Frattali, 1998, p. 245).

A third common feature of managed care systems is authorization of services. Authorization is a management technique that helps to facilitate compliance with the Federal HMO Act of 1973.

Managed care has had a tremendous impact on rehabilitation services. In the last 15 years, there has been an increase in subacute facilities to bridge the gap between acute-care hospitals and nursing facilities. Patients are discharged from acute care settings more rapidly than in previous times, necessitating the development of facilities designed to provide intermediate care and rehabilitation before a patient is discharged to a long-term care facility or home. Home health agencies also have proliferated to accommodate patients discharged to home (frequently due to caps on medical coverage).

According to Henri and Hallowell (1999), managed care challenges in speech-language pathology and audiology can be divided into five categories.

The first is consumers' **access to services:** There has been a decrease in the number of referrals from "gatekeepers" who tend to focus more on acute care. There has been an increase in lack of coverage due to clauses related to pre-existing conditions that reduce or negate the payment for rehabilitation services. Also, there is a demand from managed care organizations for consistent improvement that may not be evident in elderly patients and patients with chronic disability, multiple disabilities, or degenerative conditions. Others who have less access to services include minorities and low income individuals, as they are often not in jobs with employee health plans. In addition, some managed care organizations state that services that are provided must meet specific criteria with regard to medical necessity. Perkins and Olson (1998; as cited in Henri & Hallowell, 1999) define "medical necessity" as follows:

1. "To prevent the onset or worsening of an illness, condition, or disability;
2. To establish a diagnosis;
3. To provide palliative, curative, or restorative treatment for physical and/or mental health conditions;
4. To assist the individual to achieve or maintain maximum functional capacity in performing daily activities, taking into account both the functional capacity of the individual and those functional capacities that are appropriate for individuals of the same age" (p. 20).

Because many rehabilitation services are not considered to be medically necessary, they may not be covered under some HMOs/MCOs (Henri & Hallowell, 1999). Kahan et al. (1994, pp. 357–359), as cited by Henri and Hallowell provide some "helpful direction in supporting the medical necessity of clinical services. They present the following four criteria:

1. "The procedure must be appropriate (that is, its benefits must sufficiently outweigh its risks to make it worth performing, and it must do at least as well as the next best available procedure);
2. It would be improper care not to recommend this service;
3. There is a reasonable chance that the procedure will benefit the patient;
4. The benefit to the patient is not small" (Henri & Hallowell, p. 19).

The second category relates to the **quality, intensity, duration, and frequency of care that is provided**. Based on a particular diagnosis, the number of treatment sessions may be predetermined, with the number being restricted within a given period of time. In some cases, duration of therapy is limited to six visits in acute stages, and 60 days during rehabilitation as opposed to the more traditional 1 to 18 months for CVAs, TBIs, and those with degenerative nervous system disorders. "These restrictions also create the possibility of a circular process; when little progress is made because few visits are permitted, the insurer denies further care because little progress was made" (Henri & Hallowell, 1999, p. 7). There also may be delays in the initiation of treatment while waiting for authorization or reauthorization for services. Treatment sessions are shorter, usually lasting 30 to 45 minutes instead of the traditional 60 minutes. It is also becoming more common for insurance companies to intervene with goal writing, treatment planning, scheduling, determining progress, and selecting augmentative communication devices (Henri & Hallowell, 1999).

The **fiscal stability of service providing agencies** is the third category of managed care challenges for the speech-language pathologist or audiologist. Tied in with this is the fourth category of challenge which is the **livelihood of professionals in the field**. Slow processing of claims, and reduced coverage (sometimes up to 80% reduction in rates to members of some HMOs/MCOs) have led to reduced coverage of services and reductions in the number of staff. Some clinicians are hiring more assistants and aides as a lower cost method of providing coverage in therapy. Although trained paraprofessionals can help with some tasks, some HMOs/MCOs will not pay unless services are provided by the highest qualified provider. Some clinicians use trained volunteers and family members to assist with generalization and maintenance. There is also increased competition between agencies to become providers for specific HMOs/MCOs (Henri & Hallowell, 1999).

Approximately 30% of submissions for authorization of diagnosis and treatment are denied, although approximately 90% of the appeals result in overturning the original refusal. To appeal, the clinician needs to submit "a written request for authorization by the primary care physician or additional supporting documentation resulting from the evaluation or treatment" (Henri & Hallowell, 1999, p. 23). Additionally, the patient also can file a complaint with the human resources department where he is employed, and he should also submit a copy sent to the insurer. It is prudent to file a complaint with the state insurance commissioner if the appeal is not upheld. Wherever the complaint is filed, it is helpful to be cooperative, not adversarial, and to always be a patient advocate (Henri & Hallowell, 1999).

The **maintenance of professional integrity** is the fifth category of challenges. Members of the American Speech-Language-Hearing Association (ASHA) are bound by a Code of Ethics (2003) that helps to define and shape the reputation and worthiness of the profession.

The increased use of paraprofessionals and the increased emphasis on multitasking are direct threats to our professional integrity. The role of HMOs/MCOs in the decision-making process removes some of the professional autonomy that has long been a standard for ASHA members. Furthermore, the demand for cost-effective treatment, reducing costs, and increasing the productivity frequently puts clinicians in a moral and ethical bind. Also at issue is the provision of care to patients who cannot reasonably benefit from services in order to meet productivity requirements. The compromising of care to meet arbitrary standards set by the health care industry has a negative impact on our profession.

These challenges dictate the need for our profession to develop outcome measures that can be used to justify decision making related to the provision of diagnostic and therapeutic interventions. Donabedian (1980) defines the term "outcome" as "a change in a patient's current and future health status that can be attributed to antecedent health care." Typically, outcomes have emphasized the physical and physiologic aspects of performance. However, in the current health care environment, outcomes need to reflect changes in the social and psychological functioning of the patient as well. Other components of health which merit consideration include the patient's attitudes, his satisfaction with the services he is receiving, his health-related knowledge, and the behavioral changes that come about as a result of his knowledge and attitude.

In 1993, ASHA created a Task Force on Treatment Outcomes and Cost Effectiveness when ASHA members requested data that documented effectiveness of speech-language pathology and audiology services. Out of that initiative, a national database, The National Outcomes Measurement System (NOMS), was created in 1997. "The purpose of NOMS is to collect aggregated national outcomes data from speech-language pathologists and audiologists working with adults and children in both school and health care settings" (http://www.asha.org/members/research/NOMS retrieved 01/03/09). To facilitate and standardize the data collection, ASHA's Functional Communication Measures (FCMs) were developed. "FCMs are a series of disorder-specific, seven-point rating scales designed to describe the change in an individual's functional communication and/or swallowing ability over time." Clinicians participating in the NOMS project choose FCMs and assess the client's ability on each measure at the beginning and conclusion of treatment, thereby documenting the effectiveness of services. Data are collected on three populations:

1. adults in health care settings,
2. preschoolers in health care or school settings, and
3. children enrolled in K–12 school settings.

"It is hoped that the clinicians can use the data as measured by the Functional Communication Measures to validate their services, improve the quality of their services, and make adjustments in the practice patterns as needed" (Henri & Hallowell, 1999).

In October, 2008, NOMS showed the following results reflecting patients' responses to two statements:

1. "Overall, the SLP services were satisfactory."
   a. Strongly agree    61.7%
   b. Agree             36.0%
   c. Neutral            2.2%

2. "I believe that my communication improved because of the SLP services."
   d. Strongly agree    53.5%
   e. Agree             38.1%
   f. Neutral            7.1%
   g. Disagree           1.2%

Appendixes 2A, 2B, and 2C contain lists of the FCMs for each population in the NOMS project, and examples of the levels of ability. It should be noted that clinicians must register as a participant in the NOMS project in order to access the outcomes data. More information on how to participate in ASHA's NOMS project can be obtained from ASHA's Web site (http://www.asha.org).

ASHA has pointed out the need to collect state and national outcomes data in order to effectively lobby legislators to allocate a portion of the health care dollars to rehabilitation services such as speech-language pathology. With increased dollars come increased access for those in need of speech-language pathology and audiology services. There also is a need to compare state performances to the national averages as a "benchmark of quality of care" (Frattai, 1998, p. 37).

One also must consider the temporal aspect of outcomes.

Intermediate outcomes determine, from session to session, whether treatment is benefiting the client . . . Instrumental outcomes activate the learning process. These are outcomes that, when reached, trigger the ultimate outcome . . . Ultimate outcomes demonstrate the social or ecological validity of interventions, such as functional communication, reemployability, community reintegration, and individually defined quality of life. (Frattali, 1999, p. 39)

The Agency for Health Care Policy and Research (AHCPR) has, in the near past, worked on the development of nationally recognized clinical practice guidelines, but has recently redirected its efforts to establish evidence-based practice centers." The purpose of these centers is to "provide extensive literature review on assigned topics and to produce "evidence reports" or technology assessments so that clinicians can make critical health care decisions based upon the latest and most comprehensive scientific knowledge" (Cornett & Davison, 1999, p. 55).

Spath (1994) suggests that clinicians should concentrate on a variety of elements to achieve outcomes management. Spath maintains that outcomes management includes (1) specifying outcomes, (2) measuring outcomes, (3) designing information systems, and (4) improving the processing of information. Not only does the clinician/health care team need to define the outcomes, he or she also must specify how the attainment of the expected outcomes will be measured and documented. To that end, assessment instruments that are both valid and reliable must be developed and/or utilized. This is in keeping with ASHA's NOMS initiative.

In today's business, education, and health care environments, there is emphasis on developing and/or adapting efficient information systems, both electronic and (decreasingly) manual. Regardless of which system is adopted, it must meet the needs of the patient and the health care team in terms of everyday operations and with regard to data management (input, access, and retrieval) (Spath, 1994). Documentation should be brief and concise. It should include a brief history and a description of the presenting problem. A summary of formal and informal assessment procedures should follow. Outcome-oriented, long-range goals should be included in the report, as well as a diagnosis and prognostic statement and, if possible, the estimated duration of treatment should also be included. Session by session progress notes documenting any change of goals (including justifications), and progress toward goals in that particular session should also be noted (Henri & Hallowell, 1999).

Finally, Spath's fourth component of outcomes management is to improve the process. By this, Spath means that we must all be diligent about improving the therapeutic processes, and improving the techniques we use to accomplish the functional goals set for our patients.

## Malpractice

There are two approaches to defining malpractice in the health care professions. Traditionally, malpractice referred to conduct that constitutes professional negligence. The broader, more complete definition which fits with today's atmosphere is as follows:

Any potential legal basis for imposition of liability, including:

▓ Professional negligence;
▓ Breach of a patient-professional contractual promise;
▓ Liability for defective care-related equipment or products that injure patients or clients;
▓ Strict liability (absolute liability without regard for fault) for abnormally dangerous care-related professional activities; and
▓ Intentional care-related provider misconduct conduct (Scott, 2000, p. 4).

Negligence is the "delivery of patient care that falls below the standards expected of ordinary reasonable practitioners of the same profession acting under the same or similar circumstances" (Scott, p. 5). Should a patient file a complaint of malpractice, he must prove four requisite elements:

1. The provider owed the patient a special duty of due care;
2. The provider violated the special duty owed;
3. As a result, the patient was injured; and
4. The patient is entitled to legally recognized money damages (Scott, p. 6).

Rowland (1988) wrote that

Malpractice is not limited to the negligent (unintentional) infliction or creation of pain during evaluation or management of a disorder. Malpractice can include: (1) misdiagnosis; (2) failure to reveal alternative remediation; (3) improper or substandard remediation techniques; (4) failure to refer when not competent to manage; (5) referral to an inferior system for management; (6) breach of an actual warranty (for service or for a product); (7) breach of an implied warranty; (8) release of information to unauthorized persons (including "loose talk") or failure to release information to unauthorized persons; (9) failure to properly instruct in the use of a potentially hazardous product; (10) failure to warn of a potential hazard or harm. (p. 45)

He defined malpractice as existing "anytime a physical or mental injury or economic loss results from an action or omission which falls within a recognized standard of care" (Rowland 1988, p. 45).

ASHA also has a few cases of malpractice reported annually. Typically, these complaints are related to deceitful and/or misleading advertising, and insurance fraud. Other areas of complaint include license fraud; general practice fraud; unprofessional conduct; low standards of care; unethical practices; refusal of services; and inadequate record keeping (Trace & Breske, 1993).

To file a complaint of malpractice with ASHA, the complainer must file the complaint in writing, and it must be signed by the individual filing the grievance. The complainant also signs a waiver of confidentiality. The complaint is then sent to the violator, who has 45 days to respond. The Ethical Practices Board convenes and either dismisses or adjudicates the complaint. The Board informs the parties of their decision and, when appropriate, cites the specific code infringement, and the proposed sanction. The violator can request an appearance before the Board, and take counsel if so desired. ASHA typically has three forms of retribution: the reprimand, censure, and revocation of membership and/or certification. The reprimand is a private "slap on the wrist," whereas censure is a public "slap on the wrist." Revocation of membership and/or certification takes away the right of the person as a member of ASHA to continue practicing as a speech-language pathologist.

### Malpractice Versus Liability

Liability is the state of being responsible for the professional treatment of one's patient and to the ASHA Code of Ethics, and is the result of malpractice. Professional liability occurs when the speech-language pathologist's conduct is negligent during the course of assessing or treating a patient, and this negligence results in injury to the patient. It is difficult to define malpractice, but any treatment that causes injury to the patient, or that can be interpreted as harmful, unprofessional, or neglectful could be defined as malpractice. In essence, malpractice is the action of conduct that is unprofessional, and liability is the result.

Negligence law covers compensation of individuals who have been accidentally harmed by another. It is based on the principle of reasonable care: if your failure to use reasonable care in the treatment of your patient results in harm to that person, potentially, you could be legally liable. For that reason, it is advisable for speech-language pathologists to carry liability insurance.

## Strategies to Avoid Being the Subject of a Complaint

One of the most important strategies to avoid being the subject of a complaint is to establish positive relationships with patients and their families. This includes returning phone calls, not neglecting appointments, adhering to schedules, maintaining a pleasant attitude, and addressing the needs and concerns of the patient and/or his or her caregivers. It is also helpful to educate the patient and his or her family about the disorder or illness, and to help them establish realistic goals for the patient.

Finally, documentation is absolutely critical in avoiding becoming a violator. Documentation should include the following:

1. Date and time seen
2. Patient concerns/complaints
3. Description of visits/comments/feedback
4. Specific language regarding the disorder or illness
5. Appropriately marking errors (Trace & Breske, 1993).

Appropriately marked errors are those that have a single line drawn through the error, are labeled as an error, and have the date and the clinician's signature. Never use correction fluid on a legal document.

## Being Served a Summons

If you are served with a summons, the first course of action should be to notify your supervisor and/or legal counsel and discuss the reason for the summons. If a malpractice suit is filed, you should also contact your insurance carrier.

To avoid a default judgment, immediately prepare a response to the summons. Your attorney should file the response. Typically, there is a time limit of 30 days in which the alleged violator has to file his or her response, although this can vary from state to state.

You should work closely with your attorney and take an active role in your response and defense. This is especially critical in health care cases in which the lawyer may need some guidance in understanding the specific circumstances surrounding the alleged violation. You should review the patient's medical records, and educate your attorney accordingly.

It is advisable to attend the patient's deposition. Also, as a witness, you should explain the terminology (to help gain the jury's respect) and use demonstrative aids such as videos and audio recordings to explain the type of service being provided to the patient (Trace & Breske, 1993).

## Summary

The above information is presented in order to make the new clinician familiar with some of the more difficult decision-making situations sometimes faced by practicing clinicians. It behooves the clinician to hold "paramount" (as written in the ASHA Code of Ethics) the welfare of our patients by recognizing their needs and expectations with regards to rehabilitation or habilitation of their disabilities, impairments, and/or handicaps.

## References

American Speech-Language-Hearing Association. (1997). *National outcomes measures.* Rockville, MD: Author.

American Speech-Language-Hearing Association. (2003). *Code of ethics.* Rockville, MD: Author.

Centers for Disease Control. http://www.cdc.gov

Cornett, B. S., & Davidson, T. L. (1999). Structuring clinical practice: Guidelines, pathways, and protocols. In B. S. Cornett (Ed.), *Clinical practice management for speech-language pathologists.* Gaithersburg, MD: Aspen.

Dikengil, A. T. (1998). *Handbook of home health care for the speech-language pathologist.* San Diego, CA: Singular.

Donabedian, A. (1980). *The definition of quality and approaches to its assessment.* Ann Arbor, MI: Health Administrative Press.

Frattali, C. M. (1998). Outcomes measurement: Definitions, dimensions and perspectives. In C. Frattali (Ed.), *Measuring outcomes in speech-language pathology* (pp. 1-27). New York: Thieme.

Frattali, C. M. (1999). Measuring and managing outcomes. In B. S. Cornett (Ed.), *Clinical practice management in speech-language pathology* (pp. 29-51). Gaithersburg, MD: Aspen.

Griffin, K. M., & Fazen, M. (1993, Winter). A managed care strategy for practitioners. *Quality Improvement Digest,* pp. 1-7.

Henri, B. P., & Hallowell, B. (1999). Mastering managed care: Problems and possibilities. In B. S. Cornett (Ed.), *Clinical practice management in speech-language pathology: Principles and practicalities.* Gaithersburg, MD: Aspen.

Kahan, J. P., Bernstein, S. J., Leape, L. L., Hilborne, L. H., Park, R. E., Parker, L., et al. (1994). Measuring the necessity of medical procedures. *Medical Care, 32,* 357-365.

Perkins, J., & Olson, K. (1998). The threat of evidence-based definitions of medical necessity. *Health Advocate.* Los Angeles: National Health Law Program.

Rowland, R. C. (1988, January). Malpractice in audiology and speech-language pathology. *ASHA,* pp. 45-48.

Scott, R. W. (2000). *Legal aspects of documenting patient care* (2nd ed.). Gaithersburg, MD: Aspen.

Spath, P. (Ed.) (1994). *Clinical paths: Tools for outcomes management.* Chicago: American Hospital Publishing.

Trace, R., & Breske, S. (1993, July 19). Legal issues in speech-language pathology: Documentation and communication are key safeguards. *Advances for Speech-Language Pathologists and Audiologists.*

## APPENDIX 2A
## The 15 Functional Communication Measures in Adult Health Care Settings and 2 Examples of Level Criteria for "Spoken Language Comprehension":

a.  Alaryngeal Communication

b.  Attention

c.  Augmentative and Alternative Communication

d.  Fluency

e.  Memory

f.  Motor speech

g.  Pragmatis

h.  Problem Solving

i.  Reading

j.  Spoken Language Comprehension

k.  Spoken Language Expression

l.  Swallowing

m.  Voice

n.  Voice following tracheostomy

o.  Writing

**Level 1:**  The individual is alert but unable to follow simple directions or respond to yes/no questions, even with cues.

**Level 7:**  The individual's ability to independently participate in vocational, avocational, and social activities is not limited by spoken language comprehension. When difficulty with comprehension occurs, the individual consistently uses a compensatory strategy.

## APPENDIX 2B
## The 6 Functional Communication Measures in Pre-K Settings and 2 Examples of Level Criteria for "Spoken Language Comprehension":

1. Articulation/Intelligibility

2. Cognitive Orientation

3. Pragmatics

4. Spoken Language Comprehension

5. Spoken Language Production

6. Swallowing

**Level 1:** Child understands a limited number of common object and action labels and simple directions only in highly structured, repetitive daily routines, with consistent maximal cueing.

**Level 7:** Child's ability to participate in adult-child, peer, and group activities is not limited by language comprehension. Repetition and rephrasing are rarely required.

## APPENDIX 2C
## The 12 Functional Communication Measures in K–12 School Settings and 2 Examples of Level Criteria for "Spoken Language Comprehension":

1. Composition

2. Emergent Literacy

3. Fluency

4. Intelligibility

5. Pragmatics

6. Reading Comprehension

7. Speech Sound Production

8. Spoken Language Comprehension

9. Spoken Language Production

10. Voice

11. Word Recognition

12. Writing Accuracy

*Note:* The writers of the FCMs for the K-12 population in schools note that the FCMs "were designed to describe the change in functional communication abilities over time from entrance to dismissal from the speech-language treatment program or over the course of an IEP year" (http://www.asha.org/members/research/NOMS, retrieved 01.03.09). They further state that the attainment of the measures are based on "informal clinical observations," not standardized or other types of assessments.

## Spoken Language Production

Low Verbal Demand: Verbal initiations and responses that primarily require language content and forms acquired at a younger age than the student's current chronologic age.

High Verbal Demand: Verbal initiations and responses that primarily require language content and forms representing more recently acquired structures for the student's chronologic age.

**Level 1:** The student's verbal messages are rarely age appropriate in low verbal demand educational activities, but are never age-appropriate in high verbal-demand educational activities.

**Level 7:** The student's independent verbal messages are consistently age appropriate. The student's successful participation in educational activities is not dependent on others to provide additional support to reduce the verbal demand. The student is consistently able to use compensatory strategies when needed.

*Chapter 3*

# Universal Precautions Against Blood-Borne Pathogens and Other Potentially Infectious Material

## Introduction

In the 1970s, the National Nosocomial Infections Surveillance System (NNIS) was formed to monitor the incidence of nosocomial (health care associated, hospital-acquired) infections and associated risk factors in 300 hospitals. In 2006, the NNIS was redesigned as the National Healthcare Safety Network and is managed by the Centers for Disease Control's Division of Healthcare Quality Promotion. Incidence figures from CDC/NNIS indicate that approximately 2 million cases of nosocomial infections, also known as hospital-acquired infections (HAIs), occur annually. This figure translates to approximately 10% of all hospital patients. Of the 2 million cases, 80,000 die. To put it another way, one of every 136 patients will develop an infection while in the hospital.

Although the concept of "universal precautions" was not formally introduced by the Centers for Disease Control (CDC) until 1987, recognition of the fact that hand washing helps reduce maternal death during and immediately following childbirth was first documented in 1847. In 1961, the U.S. Public Health Service developed a film directed toward health care workers that included demonstrations of how to wash hands in a medical setting to decrease the possibility of nosocomial infections. In that film, it was recommended that individuals wash for one to two minutes with soap and water prior to and following patient contact. They indicated that rinsing with an antiseptic solution was acceptable in emergency situations or instances when there was no sink, but it was not as effective as soap and water. Comparisons of hand washing with soaps versus alcohol rubs and gels are presented later in this chapter.

However, universal precautions go beyond hand washing. Golper and Brown (2005) write that there are three primary areas of concern with regard to risk management:

1. Risks to the safety and health of employees and clients
2. Risks for legal action
3. Risks to the financial viability of the organization or agency (p. 67)

Therefore, specific policies and procedures need to be developed to address each of these areas of concern. Anytime you are providing care in a medical, residential, or educational setting, you, as the clinician, are in a position where you could pass an illness on to a patient as well as being exposed to a variety of communicable diseases. There are three primary pathways for infection:

1. Nosocomial Infections: Hepatitis B, HIV, tuberculosis, cytomegalovirus, herpes simplex, and influenza are the most prevalent exposures in a medical setting.
2. Chain of Infections: A patient may have one infection that makes him or her at increased risk for a chain of infections due to decreased immune systems.
3. Increased risk of infections in patients: Patients who have underlying disease (especially cardiopulmonary disease), pre-existing conditions (such as connective tissues diseases), and/or immunodeficiency are particularly at risk. Patients who are postoperative, particularly thoracic or abdominal surgery, or who are on chemotherapy, are also highly susceptible to HAIs. In addition, neonates and the elderly populations are more prone to nosocomial infections.

The universal precautions suggested by the Centers for Disease Control in 1987 became part of the standards of the U.S. Department of Labor Occupational Safety and Health Administration (OSHA) in 1991.

They were designed to decrease the risk of injury or illness of health-care workers who are exposed to infected patients by enhancing infection control practices (Jones, 2002). But, equally important is the need to implement universal precautions to protect our patients from infection. Hospitalized patients are at particular risk for infection due to the fact that they have weakened immune systems due to their illness and/or side-effects from various treatments.

## Blood-Borne Pathogens

Blood-borne pathogens are defined as pathogenic microorganisms that are present in human blood, human blood components, or products made from human blood that can cause disease in humans. The most prevalent pathogens include human immunodeficiency virus (HIV), hepatitis B virus (HBV), and hepatitis C virus. Other diseases can also be present. All medical personnel, as well as those working in private practices, skilled nursing facilities, and schools, should be trained annually on the prevention of diseases due to exposure to blood-borne pathogens. As part of the precautions, Bamigboye and Adesanya (2006) suggest that "under universal precautions, blood and certain body fluids of all patients are considered potentially infectious for human immuno-deficiency virus (HIV) and other blood borne pathogens" (p. 112).

### *Terminology*

Terms identified and defined as related to blood-borne pathogens by the University of Florida blood-borne pathogens task force include the following:

**Decontamination:** The use of physical or chemical means to remove, inactivate or destroy blood-borne pathogens on a surface or item to the point where they are no longer capable of transmitting infectious particles and the surface or item is rendered safe for handling, use, or disposal.

**Engineering Controls:** Controls (e.g., sharps disposal containers, self-sheathing needles) that isolate or remove the blood-borne pathogens hazard from the workplace.

**Exposure Incident:** A specific eye, mouth, or other mucous membrane, nonintact skin, or parenteral contact with blood or other potentially infectious materials that results from the performance of an employee's duties.

**Occupational Exposure:** Reasonably anticipated skin, eye, mucous membrane, or parenteral contact with blood or other potentially infectious materials that results from the performance of an employee's duties.

**Other Potentially Infectious Materials (OPIM):** Materials other than human blood are potentially infectious for blood-borne pathogens. These include (1) the following human body fluids: semen, vaginal secretions, cerebrospinal fluid, synovial fluid, pleural fluid, pericardial fluid, peritoneal fluid, amniotic fluid, saliva in dental procedures, any body fluid that is visibly contaminated with blood, and all body fluids in situations where it is difficult or impossible to differentiate between body fluids; (2) any unfixed tissue or organ (other than intact skin) from a human (living or dead); (3) HIV or HBV-containing cell or tissue cultures, organ cultures, culture medium, or other solutions; and (4) blood, organs, or other tissues from experimental animals infected with HIV or HBV.

**Parenteral:** Piercing mucous membranes or the skin barrier through such events as needlesticks, human bites, cuts, or abrasions.

**Personal Protective Equipment (PPE):** Specialized clothing or equipment worn by an employee for protection against a hazard. General work clothes (e.g., uniforms, pants, shirts, or blouses) not intended to function as protection against a hazard are not considered to be personal protective equipment.

**Universal Precautions:** An approach to infection control. According to the concept of Universal Precautions, all human blood and certain human body fluids are treated as if known to be infectious for HIV, HBV, and other blood-borne pathogens. PPE (gowns, gloves, face shields, protective eyewear, and/or aprons) should be worn to prevent skin or mucous membrane contact with blood and OPIM. Hands should be washed after each patient encounter, even if gloves have been worn.

**Work Practice Controls:** Practices that reduce the likelihood of exposure by altering the manner in which a task is performed (e.g., prohibiting recapping of needles).

## Hepatitis B and Hepatitis B Vaccine

Hepatitis B is a liver infection that is caused by the hepatitis B virus (HBV). Typically, it has a slow onset with mild symptoms that may or may not increase in severity. Typical symptoms include a vague feeling of impending illness, loss of appetite, extreme tiredness, nausea with or without vomiting, stomach pain, dark urine, and jaundice. Some patients demonstrate skin rashes and joint pain as well.

Hepatitis B can be caused by many different scenarios:

1. Unprotected sexual contact with an infected person
2. Sharing needles with an infected person
3. Occupational exposures including needle sticks or other body fluid exposures
4. Household contact with a person who has either an acute infection or is a chronic carrier of certain blood products
5. Hemodialysis

However, it should be noted that about 33% of individuals with active hepatitis do not have readily identified risk factors. There is a vaccine (Heptavax B) that is delivered by 3 shots over a 6-month period. Any time over the first 6 months following the completion of the series of vaccinations, one should have antibody testing to ensure that the individual is protected.

HBV has an incidence figure of approximately 300,000 persons a year. Typically, these are young adults, and over 12,000 are health care workers. It is also possible to become a chronic carrier, which means the HBV is in their blood for more than 6 months. During this time it is possible to spread the infection to others, particularly if one develops a disease known as "chronic active hepatitis."

Individuals infected with HBV have an increased (12–30 times) risk of developing liver cancer when compared to the uninfected population. A fatality rate of 1.4% (approximately 4,000 persons annually) is documented. There is no specific treatment and no cure for Hepatitis B.

## Human Immunodeficiency Virus/Acquired Immunodeficiency Syndrome (HIV/AIDS)

HIV was first recognized by the Centers for Disease Control in 1981. HIV decreases the body's ability to fight infection by destroying what is known as CD4 (T-cell) lymphocytes. T-cells are groups of white blood cells that protect the body from bacteria, viruses, and other germs. When the HIV has significantly decreased the body's defense mechanisms, and the "number of normal CD4 cells drops below the threshold level needed to defend the body against infections, the person develops AIDS" (Harvard Health Publications, 2007, p. 2). HIV is spread through contact with body fluids, especially blood, semen, and vaginal secretions.

> HIV particles invade CD4 lymphocytes and use the cells' own genetic materials to produce billions of new HIV particles. These new particles cause the infected CD4 cells to burst (lyse). The new particles can then enter the bloodstream and infect other cells. (Harvard Health Publications, 2007, p. 2)

The individual with HIV has an increased risk of infection and a higher risk of contracting some cancers.

Most settings require their employees to be retrained in universal precautions and blood-borne pathogens on a yearly basis. If an individual's position/job changes in the course of a year, it may be deemed necessary that the employee retake the course even if it has not been a year since the last training.

## What Should Be in Training?

Again drawing from the Environmental Health and Safety department at the University of Florida, the following topics should be addressed in training on blood-borne pathogens:

1. Providing a copy of the blood-borne pathogen standards.
2. A general explanation of the epidemiology and symptoms of bloodborne diseases.
3. An explanation of modes of transmission of blood-borne pathogens.
4. A review of the exposure control plan.

5. An explanation of the appropriate methods for recognizing procedures and other activities that may involve exposure to blood and OPIM.
6. An explanation of the use and limitations of practices that will prevent or reduce the likelihood of exposure. This includes the appropriate use of personal protective equipment and proper work practices.
7. Information on the types, proper use, location, removal, handling, decontamination, and/or disposal of personal protective equipment.
8. An explanation of the rationale for selecting personal protective equipment.
9. Information on the hepatitis B vaccine, including information on its efficacy, safety, and the benefits of being protected against hepatitis B.
10. An explanation of the postexposure evaluation in the event of an exposure including reporting mechanisms, time frames for reporting, and the medical management that is available.
11. Information on the management of emergencies associated with bloodborne pathogens including persons to contact and precautions.
12. Review of signs, labeling, and bagging procedures associated with prevention and control of blood-borne pathogen.

## Universal Precautions

Universal precautions/infection control is comprised of five primary components: (1) risk management, (2) setting of standards and protocols, (3) risk reduction, (4) postexposure measures, and (5) first aid. Numerous measures can be taken to promote a safe work environment. In the *Encyclopedia of Nursing and Allied Health*, the following measures are suggested:

1. education of employees about occupational risks and methods of prevention of HIV and other infectious diseases;
2. provision of protective equipment;
3. provision of appropriate disinfectants to clean up spills of blood or other body fluids;
4. easy accessibility of puncture resistant sharps containers;

5. maintaining appropriate staffing levels;
6. measures that reduce and prevent stress, isolation, and burnout;
7. controlling shift lengths;
8. providing postexposure counseling, treatment, and follow-up.

In addition, the Centers for Disease Control recommend vaccinations against hepatitis B virus, flu, measles, mumps, rubella, and tetanus.

## Personal Protective Equipment (PPE)

Personal protective equipment includes gloves, gowns, laboratory coats, face shields, face masks, eye protection, foot coverings, resuscitation bags, and other such items. They should be provided by the employer in order to prevent exposure of the employees and patients to blood-borne pathogens or OPIM. Not all items will be used with every patient, but it falls on the employee to determine which PPE is most appropriate for the setting and patient. PPE is designed to prohibit the passage of blood or OPIM to the employee's skin, street clothes, or mucous membranes.

## Housekeeping

Housekeeping refers to cleaning, disinfection, and sterilization practices that should be practiced by everyone with patient contact. Blood spills and OPIM spills must be decontaminated with a 1:10 dilution of household bleach. Work surfaces should be cleaned and disinfected with a 1:100 dilution of household bleach. There are other disinfectants on the market, but they only should be used if they are labeled as "tuberculocidal." The 1:10 dilution should not be stored but should be mixed fresh each day. Contaminated areas should be covered with the bleach solution and then wiped down with paper towels. Gloves and other PPE as appropriate should be worn when decontaminating a work area. The solution should remain on the item being cleaned for 10 minutes.

Contaminated linens should be managed using standard universal precautions that are described throughout this chapter.

## Labels

Red bags, red containers, or warning labels should be used with all contaminated items. The labels should be fluorescent orange or orange-red, and should include the biohazard symbol.

Warning labels should be affixed to any containers of regulated waste materials, including refrigerators and freezers where blood and other hazardous or infectious materials are stored.

## Exposure Prevention

Employees should observe universal precautions and engineering and work practice controls to eliminate or at least minimize risks of exposure. This includes wearing personal protective equipment. Again referencing the guidelines at the University of Florida, engineering controls include the following:

1. Provision and maintenance of hand washing facilities with adequate supplies. The antibacterial gels are considered to be just as effective (if not more effective) than hand washing. Hand-gel dispensers should be in all patient's rooms and all examination, treatment, and operating rooms.
2. Hand washing shall be performed after removal of gloves and after contact with blood or OPIM.
3. Employees who have exudative lesions or weeping dermatitis shall refrain from handling blood or OPIM until the condition resolves.
4. Contaminated sharps and needles shall not be bent, recapped, or sheared.
5. Contaminated sharps and needles shall be disposed of in puncture resistant, color-coded, or labeled, leak-proof containers.
6. Eating, drinking, smoking, handling contact lenses, and applying cosmetics are prohibited in work areas where there is a potential for blood or OPIM exposure.
7. Food and drink are prohibited in work areas where there is a potential for blood or OPIM exposure.

8. All procedures involving blood and OPIM shall be performed in such a manner to minimize splashing, spraying, spattering, generation of droplets, or aerosolization of these substances.
9. Mouth pipetting and suctioning are not allowed.
10. Resuscitation devices including mouthpieces or resuscitation bags shall be available for use in areas where the need for resuscitation is predictable.
11. All specimens of blood or OPIM shall be placed in closable, leak-proof containers prior to transport. If contamination of the outside of the primary container is likely, then a second container such as a plastic bag should be placed over the primary container to prevent contamination and/or leakage during handling, storage, or transport.

## Exposure Management

Skin and wound exposures should be washed immediately with soap and water. The incident should be reported to the immediate supervisor. The exposed individual should have medical follow-up no later than 24 hours postevent. Notes on the evaluation and follow-up are considered confidential. Follow-up should contain the following:

1. Documentation of the route and circumstances of the exposure
2. Identification of the source individual should be documented unless it is unfeasible or prohibited by state law.
3. The source should be tested for HIV or HBV. If the source has already been identified as having HIV or HBV, retesting is not necessary. The results of that testing will be disclosed to the affected employee.
4. Serologic testing of the exposed employee shall be offered within the provisions of law regarding HIV. If the employee consents to baseline blood collection, but chooses not to be tested for HIV at that time, the sample shall be held for 90 days after the incident enabling the employee to have HIV testing within 90 days.

The evaluations and follow-up protocols are based on the U.S. Public Health Service recommendations. A written follow-up letter shall be provided to the exposed employee within 15 days of the completion of the evaluation. The letter shall document:

1. That the employee has been informed of the results of the evaluation.
2. That the employee has been informed about any medical conditions resulting from exposure to blood or other potentially infectious materials, which require any further evaluation or treatment.
3. The hepatitis B immunization status and the need for immunization.
4. The letter shall not include any confidential material.

The medical personnel responsible for evaluation of exposures shall be knowledgeable about the OSHA Blood-borne Pathogen standard 1910.1030, and state statutes. The evaluating agency shall provide the results of the source individual's blood testing and the immunization status to the medical evaluator. A description of the exposed employee's duties as they relate to the incident shall also be given to the evaluator.

Furthermore, exposure Control Plans should be reviewed and updated annually to reflect the latest standards regarding blood-borne pathogens and OPIM.

## Special Concerns Related to Speech-Language Pathology

Some universal precautions have more applicability to speech-language pathologists working in outpatient clinics and other nonhospital settings and should be adhered to at all times. One of these is the appropriate use of personal protective equipment (PPE). Speech-language pathologists should wear gloves during the following activities:

1. oral-facial exam
2. middle ear testing
3. handling or fabricating ear molds and other prostheses
4. swallowing assessments and therapy
5. assessment of laryngeal functioning
6. assessment of respiratory functioning
7. impedance probe tips
8. otoscopic specula

Speech-language pathologists also should be cognizant of appropriate cleaning, sterilization, and disinfection techniques for assessment and treatment equipment ranging from tabletops and chairs, to toys, to flexible endoscopic tools. Hearing related items such as otoscopes, ear tips, earmolds on hearing aids, and impedance probe tips also need cleaning after each use. Sterilization "can be done by use of a steam autoclave, dry heat oven, chemical vapor sterilization, or immersion in a chemical sterilant for 10 hours" (Lubinski in Lubinski, & Frattali, 2001, p. 369).

## Hand Washing

Formal written guidelines on hand washing practices in hospitals were issued by CDC in 1975 and 1985. They recommended that health care workers wash between patient contacts with non-antimicrobial soap. According to CDC at that time, when tending to high-risk patients or doing invasive procedures, health care workers should wash with antimicrobial soap before and after these interactions. Still, waterless antiseptic agents were not preferred if sinks were available.

In 1995 to 1996, CDC's Healthcare Infection Control Practice Advisory Commission (HICPAC), in collaboration with other agencies, recommended the use of waterless antiseptic agents or antimicrobial soap when leaving patients' rooms. These guidelines were expansions of the previous ones that they made. Furthermore, they recommended expansion of the guidelines to other clinical settings (i.e., therapy settings, outpatient clinics). Nonetheless, compliance remained low in all settings.

There are several considerations when addressing "hand hygiene" among health care workers. Some relate to how to wash the hands, while others refer to general guidelines. Amongst the general guidelines, the following are recommended:

1. Avoid the use of artificial fingernails and fingernail extenders.
2. Trim natural fingernails to less than ¼" long.
3. Wear gloves when the potential for contact for blood or other OPIM, mucous membranes, or broken skin exists.
4. Remove gloves after working with a patient. Wash hands upon removal of gloves. Dispose of gloves upon removal.

5. If moving from a contaminated body section to a noncontaminated body section of a patient, change gloves.

Lubinski and Frattali (2001) list the following guidelines as to when speech-language pathologists should wash hands (Lubinski & Frattali, 2001; ASHA, 1989).

Upon arrival at work

Immediately, if they are potentially contaminated with blood or body fluids

Between patients

After removing gloves

Before and after handling in-patient care devices

Before preparing or serving food

Before and after performing any personal body function

When hands are obviously soiled, such as after a sneeze, nose blowing, using the bathroom

Before leaving your work setting

For isolation patients; before removing gown and mask; after removing gown and mask.

There are many guidelines that outline the appropriate and necessary steps in hand washing (Lubinski & Frattali, 2001; ASHA, 1989); Palmer, M., (1984). A compilation is below:

Remove all jewelry from hands and arms

Obtain paper towel from dispenser

Slightly lean forward over sink and avoid touching sink

Turn on water to comfortably warm level

Wet hands and forearms

Apply liquid antiseptic soap

Vigorously wash hands, wrists, and forearms for 30 to 60 seconds

Thoroughly rinse forearms, wrists, and hands

Dry hands, then wrist and forearm using a paper towel

Avoid rubbing hands too hard to create chapping

Use clean paper towel to turn off the faucet if foot or electronic controls are not available

Dispose of all paper towels in an appropriate container

Use emollient to decrease the risk of skin cracking.

Hands should be washed when they are visibly soiled, after physical contact with a patient, after removal of gloves, after touching surfaces in a patient's area, and before or after touching a patient and/or items in his or her area.

Recent studies show that the alcohol-based hand rubs are more effective than hand washing with plain soap and water, or with antimicrobial soaps and water. Reports on how much hand rub is enough are varied. However, a general guideline is "if hands feel dry after rubbing hands together for 10 to 15 seconds, an insufficient volume of product likely was applied (Boyce & Pittet, 2002, p. 13). Hand rubs that are alcohol based are the most effective agents for reducing the amount of bacteria on the hands of patients and health care personnel. These come in the form of rubs or gels; rubs are preferred over gels when available. These agents should contain at least 60% ethanol or isopropanol; the more the better. The next most effective agents are antiseptic detergents and soaps. Non-antimicrobial soaps are the least effective agents.

Alcohol towelettes have not been demonstrated as being more effective than soap and water. Also, rinses may be more effective than gels (Kramer, Rudolph, Kampf, & Pittet, 2002). Although various antiseptic agents exist (chlorhexidine, iodine compounds, idophors, phenol derivatives, and tricolsan), alcohol seems to be the best (Boyce & Pittet, 2002).

Because frequent hand washing, whether with soap and water or an alcohol-based rub, can result in drying and/or irritation of the skin, it is recommended that lotions be readily available for health care workers who must frequently wash their hands in order to maintain their own and their patients' health.

## Summary

There are three goals of infection control: (1) have all employees and volunteers immunized against preventable diseases, (2) define precautions that can prevent exposure to infectious agents, and (3) restrict exposure of health care workers to an infectious agent. To that end, universal precautions were developed. Many states and private agencies have regulations with regard to blood-borne pathogens and OPIM and will require periodic instruction in this area in order to continue to be licensed to practice. Policies and procedures are in place in most settings to advise those working with medically compromised individuals how to avoid contracting diseases and illnesses due to blood-borne pathogens and OPIM. However, a procedure is worthwhile only if it is fully implemented by those for whom it was designed to protect. In his book, *Better: A Surgeon's Notes on Performance*, Atul Gawande (2007) wrote the following:

> Stopping the epidemics spreading in our hospitals is not a problem of ignorance—of not having the know-how about what to do. It is a problem of compliance—a failure of an individual to apply that know-how correctly. (p. 22)

The ASHA Code of Ethics states that we must hold paramount the welfare of our patients. This certainly would include adhering to the guidelines designed to prevent the spread of infection from patients to each other, and from us to our patients. In an interview with A. U. Bankaitis for his article, Infection Control, Mosheim (2005) quotes her as saying, "It is the legal and ethical responsibility of clinicians to ensure that appropriate infection control measures are in place and practiced consistently." The very lives of our patients, and potentially, ourselves, can be threatened if universal precautions are not heeded.

## References

ASHA. (1989). AIDS/HIV: Implications for speech-language pathologists and audiologists. *Asha, 29*, 33–37.

Bamigboye, A. P., & Adesanya, A. T. (2006). Knowledge and practice of universal precautions among qualifying medical and nursing students: A case of Obafemi Awolowo University Teaching Hospitals Complex, ILE-IFE. *Research Journal of Medicine and Medical Sciences, 1*(3), 112–116.

Boyce, J. M., & Pittet, D. (2002). The guideline for hand hygiene in health-care settings. *Morbidity and Mortality Weekly Report, 51*(RR-16), 1–45.

Centers for Disease Control Healthcare Infection Control Practices Advisory Committee 9HICPAC). (n.d.) *Hand hygiene guidelines.* www.cdc.gov/mmwr/PDF/rr/rr5116.pdf

Encyclopedia of Nursing and Allied Health. (05/09/2001). *Universal precautions.* Available from: Health.enotes.com/nursing-encyclopedia/universal precautions

Gawande, A. (2007). *Better: A surgeon's notes on performance.* New York: Picador of Metropolitan Books, Henry Holt and Company.

Golper, L. C, & Brown, J. E. (Eds.). (2005). *Business matters: A guide for speech-language pathologists.* Rockville, MD: American Speech-Language-Hearing Association.

Harvard Health Publications. (03/09/07). *Health A–Z.* Copyright 2006 by President and Fellows of Harvard College.

Jones, C. A. L. (2002). *Gale encyclopedia of medicine.* Detroit, MI: The Gale Group.

Kramer, A., Rudolph, P., Kampf, G., & Pittet, D. (2002). Limited efficacy of alcohol-based hand gels. *Lancet, 359,* 1489–1490.

Lubinski, R., & Frattali, C. (2001). *Professional issues in speech-language pathology and audiology* (2nd ed.). San Diego, CA: Singular.

Mosheim, J. (2005). Infection control. *Advance for Speech-Language Pathologists and Audiologists, 15*(15).

Palmer, M. (1984). *Infection control: A policy and procedure manual.* Philadelphia: W. B. Saunders.

University of Florida. (2006). *2006 Bloodborne pathogen program exposure control policy.* Gainesville, FL: Environmental Health and Safety, Biological Safety Office.

# Chapter 4

# Case Law That Had Implications for Speech-Language Pathologists in School-Based Settings

There are several instances of case law that have had implications for speech-language pathologists. In this section, six of those cases are reviewed.

## The Ann Arbor Decision: Social Dialects (1979)

### *Background Information*

The parents of the black children at Martin Luther King, Jr. Elementary School in Ann Arbor, Michigan were concerned that their Black English dialect created a barrier to their children's educational progress (their learning to read, in particular). The job of the court was to decide whether the Ann Arbor School District was violating Sec. 1703(f) "which requires educational agencies to remove all language barriers that impede children's equal participation in educational programs."

## The Players

The plaintiffs were the parents of Black children at an elementary school in Ann Arbor, Michigan. Judge Joiner of the U.S. District Court in Michigan oversaw the case.

## The Issue

The case addressed the issue (and subsequently proved) that teacher rejection of the "home language" causes student rejection of efforts in learning and such students do poorly and/or fail. A second issue was based on the observation that most teachers were perceiving the Black English dialect as errors or as indicating inferior linguistic or intellectual systems. The plaintiffs were petitioning the court to require the school district to adopt a policy whereby teachers would become more sensitive to these dialects when teaching Standard English.

## The Legal Process

The case was heard by the United States District Court in Michigan in 1979.

## The Rulings

The judgment supported this petition by ruling that the teachers were not likely to be successful in overcoming these problems without expert professional guidance, and that the school board did indeed fail to provide such guidance. The court ordered the Ann Arbor schools to develop a plan to help teachers identify speakers of Black English. It also required a plan to teach Standard English to dialect speakers, while making the teachers more sensitive to dialectal variations.

The judge also ruled that black children were, indeed, having academic problems that were compounded by teachers' insensitivity to native dialects, and especially to Black English. He stated that Black English is a rule-governed linguistic system, not disordered Standard English.

The case established a legal precedent for other schools and hoped that these schools would also recognize the linguistic validity of social dialects. It was a significant case in recognizing a long struggle to legitimize the notion of Black English in our country. What was hoped for as a result of this was that this knowledge would be used to identify and assist in responding to the needs of these children to learn.

Speech-language pathologists and other professionals in the field saw this case as a precedent establishing ruling in that it provided legal recognition of the legitimacy of Black English (Bountress, 1987).

## Impacts of the Rulings

The biggest impact the Ann Arbor case had on professionals in the speech-language pathology field was that the issue of dialects, and particularly non-standard English dialects such as Black English was recognized and widely publicized. Identifying the problem is the first step in a long process to overcome the misinterpretation of social dialects. In reality, the courts cannot legislate sensitivity to teachers, nor can they develop more educational programs. A subject such as this requires commitment at all levels of the educational system to develop positive and constructive attitudes toward minority populations. A sure way to accomplish the development of a constructive attitude is to incorporate training about dialectal and cultural differences into the university curricula for education and health-related professionals.

Certainly, the most knowledgeable of the overlapping fields of linguistics, teaching, and speech-language pathology would be the speech-language pathologist. The ruling in the case may have been enhanced if a speech-language pathologist had been consulted. A speech-language pathologist may assist teachers in identifying those children with normal dialectical differences as well as setting up interventions and training programs.

Needless to say, the Ann Arbor decision did bring the problem to attention, and although it faded quickly, it has made professionals more aware of the problems of dialect differences and hopefully made social dialects more identifiable. This case set the precedent for speech-language pathologists to work with dialect issues in the public schools.

# Rowley v. Hendrick Hudson School District: The Rowley Standard (1982)

## Background Information

The Education for All Handicapped Children Act (P.L. 94-142) provides that, in order to qualify for federal support, the state must have a policy "that assures all handicapped children the right to a free appropriate public education (FAPE)." The act also stipulated that IEPs must be written for each child receiving special education or related services in the schools. The IEP (individualized education plan) was to be the vehicle by which the FAPE is tailored to the handicapped child's unique needs.

The Rowley case was based on the word "appropriate," a subjective and vague term. The Rowley case was the first case heard by the United States Supreme Court that addressed any aspect of the EAHCA, with the issue being, what does the term "appropriate" mean?

## The Players

Amy Rowley was a deaf student at Furnace Woods School in Hendrick Hudson Central School District in Peeksill, New York. Amy was profoundly deaf with only minimal residual hearing. She was an excellent lipreader. Mr. and Mrs. Rowley, Amy's parents, were also deaf. The defendant was The School Board of the Hendrick Hudson Central School District in Peekskill, New York.

## The Preliminaries

Before Amy was placed in kindergarten, several meetings were held between the school administrators and Mr. and Mrs. Rowley to discuss Amy's school placement. It was decided that she would have a trial placement in a regular kindergarten class during which time it would be determined what supplemental services would be needed.

Several members of the school staff took sign language courses, and the office installed a teletype machine in order to facilitate communication with Mr. and Mrs. Rowley.

During the trial period, an interpreter was assigned to Amy for a two-week period. At the end of that time, the interpreter stated that Amy did not need the services of an interpreter in order to benefit from her educational setting. It was also decided that she would be fitted with an FM hearing aid.

Amy completed kindergarten, and an IEP for the next year was written. It was decided she would be placed in a regular first grade class, with an FM hearing aid. A tutor for the deaf would provide one hour of intervention per day, and she would attend speech therapy for three hours per week.

## The Issue

Mr. and Mrs. Rowley also wanted a sign-language interpreter. This had not been included on the IEP (request denied) based on (1) the interpreter's recommendation after the trial period in kindergarten, and (2) the school administration's recommendation based on their consultation with the district's Commission on the Handicapped who got expert advice from Amy's teachers and others familiar with Amy's academic and social progress.

## The Legal Process

Mr. and Mrs. Rowley requested a hearing before an independent examiner. The examiner heard evidence from both sides and agreed with the school administrators that because Amy was achieving educationally, academically, and socially without the interpreter, it was not necessary to assign one to her.

The Rowley's appealed to the New York Commission on Education who upheld the decision. The Rowley's then went to the U.S. District Court for the Southern District of New York on the basis that the denial of an interpreter violated the intent of "free appropriate public education." At this hearing, the judge found Amy to be performing better than the average child in her classroom, advancing easily from grade to grade, well-adjusted, and had "extraordinary rapport" with her teachers and peers. They also stated that Amy was not learning as much as she would if she were not deaf; thus, there was a disparity between her actual achievement and her true potential. This differential was used to define whether an appropriate education was being provided, and presumably the District Court assumed that the federal courts had full responsibility for defining "appropriate education."

The United States Court of Appeals for the Second Court affirmed the District Court's decision in a divided vote.

The U.S. Supreme Court found that, contrary to the conclusions of the lower courts, the act does define "free appropriate public education" (FAPE). The lower courts were wrong in saying that the statute requires states to maximize the handicapped child's potential "commensurate with the opportunity provided to other children." The role of the federal government is not intended to be one that mandates how states are told to educate a deaf child. FAPE required "educational instruction specially designed to meet the unique needs of the handicapped child, supported by such services as are necessary to permit the child to 'benefit' from the instruction," and that the handicapped child must have the learning capacity to benefit from special education to be eligible. Specifically, they said that educators must provide "personalized instruction with sufficient support services to permit the child to benefit educationally from the instruction."

An additional finding by the court was that parents, no matter how well motivated, do not have a right under the EAHCA to compel a school district to provide a specific program or employ a specific methodology in providing for the education of their handicapped child. In this case, an interpreter is not required, but could be in other cases where the factual circumstances were different. The courts usually will defer to educational agencies' discretion and reasonable judgment.

EAHCA placements do not have to provide the best possible education for a handicapped child without regard for expense. They do have to provide for an educational setting from which the child can benefit.

States certainly can adopt additional regulations to attempt to maximize the potential of the children with handicaps, impairments, and/or disabilities, but by federal law they must only (1) comply with the procedural guidelines of the EAHCA, and (2) develop IEPs that will enable children to benefit educationally. There were three dissenting votes by justices who felt that potential maximization was the intent of the EAHCA. The lower courts were basing their decision on the "potential maximization standard" whereas the Supreme Court based its decision on the "Basic Floor of Opportunity standard."

# Diana v. State Board of Education of California (1970)

## Background Information

This case dealt with the incorrect labeling of children from national origin minority groups. The children in this case were Mexican-American children who were being placed in classes for educable mentally retarded (EMR) children. It was pointed out that the EMR classes contained twice the number of Mexican-American students than should have been expected for the ratio of these students in the general school population.

## The Players

The parents of Diana were suing the California State Board of Education.

## The Issue

The Mexican-American children had been identified through the use of intelligence tests given in English (although their primary language was Spanish), and placed in EMR classrooms. There were a disproportionate number of Mexican-American children in these classes as a result (Howe, 1981). The case called for two changes: (1) test children in their primary language, and (2) develop interim programs for the pupils who would be taken out of EMR programs as a result of the retesting as ordered by the court (Bunnello & Sage, 1979).

When Mexican-American children were allowed to respond in Spanish to the questions on the IQ tests, they gained an average of 15 points on their scores.

## The Legal Process

Actually, this case never made it to the courts.

## The Conclusions

The decision in this case led to the development of test instruments and procedures that were appropriate for non-English-speaking children in California as well as other areas with non-English-speaking populations. Diana v. State Board of Education of California, along with other early court cases that dealt with placing groups of children into special education programs who did not belong there, such as Larry P. v. Riles and Ruiz v. State Board of Education "provided, in part, the basis for federal and state policy concerning education of the handicapped child" (Bricker, 1986, p. 107).

> The consent decree allowed non-Anglo children to choose the language in which they would respond, banned the use of verbal sections of the test, and required state psychologists to develop an IQ test appropriate for Mexican-American and other non-English speaking students. Soon after, the California state legislature passed a law requiring that test scores used for placement must be substantiated through an evaluation of the student's developmental history, cultural background, and academic achievement (Author unknown: Source, ERIC Clearinghouse on Test Measurement and Evaluation).

## Larry P. v. Wilson Riles (1972)

### Background Information

This case initially was filed in 1972 and went to trial on October 11, 1977. The judgment was entered for the parents in October 1979. The case went through numerous appeals, ultimately being heard by the U. S. Court of Appeals in 1984 where the judged ruled that Wilson Riles did not discriminate against Black children.

The primary issue in Larry P. v. Wilson Riles was that students were being placed in EMR classes on the basis of IQ tests. The defense attorneys argued that there was a racial imbalance in the numbers of black students in EMR classrooms and that it was not due to test bias. Rather, the placement should be acceptable because the parents have to provide consent for the placement. However, the court rejected the defense's argument because it believed that the parents would be influenced by the test scores.

### The Players

The plaintiff was Larry P., and the defendant was Wilson Riles, California State Public Instruction Superintendent. The judge on this case was Judge Peckham.

## *The Issue*

The case was initiated as an appeal for protection against discrimination of black children with regard to IQ tests. Due to IQ testing from 1968 to 1977, Black children had been over-represented in EMR classes. These classes were not designed to return students to the regular education classes; rather, their primary purpose was to teach "social adjustment and economic usefulness."

A pioneer developer of IQ tests in the USA stated that IQ tests were culturally biased and as such not valid for black persons. They were designed to eliminate gender bias, but not cultural bias. Judge Peckham posed the question, "What do IQ tests actually measure?" but decided not to get into the controversy about the validity of IQ tests. Rather, he said, "We will assume that the tests can accurately measure the mental ability of white children placed in EMR classes, and ask if the tests utilized for EMR placement have been validated for Black children" (Fischer & Sorenson, 1985, p. 107).

Specifically, the case examined the WISC, the WISC-R, and the Stanford-Binet.

## *The Legal Process*

The case was heard in a Federal District Court. Specifically, it was the U.S. District Court for the Northern District of California.

## *The Rulings*

Throughout the history of tests, it had never been proven that these tests were valid for black children. The use of culturally biased tests with Black children violated state and federal laws guaranteeing equal protection. Schools need to demonstrate that tests fairly show mental handicaps in Black children, and that these students are tested and placed in nondiscriminatory ways. Therefore, Judge Peckham placed the burden of proving that the tests were not discriminatory on the school officials and, of course, they could not do that (Fischer, Kelly, & Schimmel, 1981).

Judge Peckham also ruled that when a child is assigned to an EMR class, he is denied the necessary academic skills. Furthermore, he found that the defendant was not utilizing the required variety of information in making EMR placement decisions. School records lacked sufficient information about behavior, socioeconomic status, and educational background.

## PARC v. Pennsylvania (1972)

### *Background Information*

In 1954, Chief Justice Earl Warren wrote that (1) "separate but equal is not equal with regard to education" due to stigma associated with the lack of cross-cultural interaction (Rothstein, p. 12), and (2) desegregation in the schools must occur with "all deliberate speed" (Fischer et al., 1981, p. 236). Brown v. the Board of Education was the defining court case with regard to racial desegregation in public schools. It was a reversal of the 1896 U.S. Supreme Court ruling in Plessy v. Ferguson that upheld the laws of segregation as being constitutional.

PARC v. Pennsylvania was an extension of Brown v. the Board of Education, only the plaintiffs were arguing the same principle should be applied to children with handicaps, not just to children of minority races.

### *The Players*

The plaintiffs were members of the Pennsylvania Association for Retarded Citizens (PARC). The defendant was the Board of Education of the State of Pennsylvania.

### *The Issue*

The members of PARC had two goals with this case: (1) the rights of a handicapped children to receive a free education, and (2) the desire to be guaranteed education with the right for parents and the children to play an active role in determining the specifics of the training (school accountability). Pennsylvania schools had programs for the mentally handicapped, but loopholes in the law meant that some severely mentally handicapped children (mental ages lower than five years) went without any education at all.

## *The Legal Process*

This case was heard in a U.S. District Court.

## *The Rulings*

The rulings in PARC v. Pennsylvania were extremely instrumental in opening the gates to the passage of Public Law 94-142 (Education for All Handicapped Children Act) in 1975. The court mandated free public education for mentally handicapped children, and mandated evaluations for both the children recognized as mentally handicapped, and those who did not meet the criteria of being classified as mentally handicapped. Evaluations were to occur twice a year.

The court also required schools to hold due process hearings upon request, and required school officials to be accountable for placements of mentally handicapped children.

The concept of "least restrictive environment" (LRE) was suggested, but not mandated; however, it did give mainstreaming an approval from the judiciary.

A summation of the findings was written as follows: "It is the commonwealth's obligation to place each mentally retarded child in a free, public program of education and training appropriate to the child's capacity" (Rothstein, 1990, p. 101).

## Mills v. Board of Education (1972)

## *Background Information*

Mills v. Board of Education followed the PARC case, expanding on the concept of due process. Also, rather than limiting the handicaps to mental retardation, the plaintiffs were seeking to obtain the right of free and appropriate education for children with all types of handicaps.

## The Players

This suit was brought against Washington, D.C., the Department of Human Services, and the mayor. "Mills" consisted of parents and guardians of seven handicapped children in the District of Columbia.

## The Issue

All seven children were not being provided with free public education. The children were being denied equal protection and due process that are guaranteed under the 14th Amendment

## The Rulings

The plaintiffs won this case, and the defendants were ordered to provide all children with free education and also to provide within one month a list of all children being denied education. They were setting the stage for a constitutional right to special education because states provide education. The defendants did not comply with the ruling, and the case was brought to District Court again. The judge decreed that any child being denied an education was being denied his rights of due process and equal protection under the law.

This case set a procedural framework incorporated into EAHCA based on the precedent that all children, no matter what their handicapping condition, have the right to free and appropriate education. They set out an elaborate framework for what due process would entail, stating that it included labeling, placement, and exclusionary stages of decision making. Specifically, due process was to include (1) the right to a hearing with representation, (2) the right to appeal, (3) the right to have access to records, and (4) the right to written notices at all stages of the process (Rothstein, 1990, p. 3).

Finally, the district court addressed funding issues in the ruling as follows:

> If sufficient funds are not available to finance all of the services and programs that are needed and desirable in the system then the available funds must be expended equitably in such a manner that no child is entirely excluded from a publicly supported education consistent with his needs and ability to benefit there from. (Rothstein, p. 101)

# Cruzan v. Director, Missouri Department of Health (1990)

## *Background Information*

Cruzan v. Director, Missouri Department of Health (1990) was a critical case in decision making about life-sustaining treatment.

## *The Players*

The plaintiffs were the parents of a 25-year-old woman who had sustained a significant head injury in a car accident. Cruzan was subsequently diagnosed as being in a chronic vegetative state with essentially no chance of regaining her mental abilities.

## *The Issue*

Cruzan did not leave any advance directives regarding the use of life-sustaining measures. Her parents requested that artificial nutrition and hydration be discontinued, but the hospital refused to do so without a court order.

## *The Rulings*

The local court's approval was overturned by the Missouri Supreme Court and eventually upheld by the United States Supreme Court. The ruling of the Missouri Supreme Court "took an important first step by guaranteeing the right of a competent person to refuse unwanted medical treatment" (Gottlich, 1990, p. 663). The ruling of the United States Supreme Court was slightly different in that it ruled that, under certain circumstances, it extended the right to refuse treatment to incompetent persons. However, since Nancy Cruzan had left no instructions regarding her wishes, the United States Supreme Court upheld the ruling of the lower court. This ruling led to the development of advance directives, the establishment of surrogate status (allowing a competent person designated by the individual to make decisions should the individual become incompetent), additional safeguards, and the establishment of a Guardian ad Litem to act on the patient's behalf.

## Summary

Although case law never has the impact that most federal legislations carry, these cases helped lay the groundwork for the future with regard to the education of children with dialectal differences and for children who have handicapping conditions. There are so many cases that have addressed education for children with delays, disorders, and differences that it is impossible within the scope of this book to address them all. Readers are encouraged to use the references to find other cases that have had an impact on how we assess and treat children in the public schools.

## References

Bountress, N. G. (1987). The Ann Arbor decision: Implications for the speech-language pathologist. *Asha, 25*(9).

Bricker, D. D. (1986). *Early education of at-risk and handicapped infants, toddlers, and preschool children.* Glenview, IL: Scott Foresman.

Bunnello, L. C., & Sage, D. D. (1979). *Leadership and change in special education.* Englewood Cliffs, NJ: Prentice-Hall.

Fischer, L., Kelly, C., & Schimmel, D. (1981). *Teachers and the law.* New York: Longman.

Fischer, L., & Sorenson, G. P. (1985). *School law for counselors, psychologists, and social workers.* New York: Longman.

Howe, C. E. (1981). *Administration of special education.* Denver, CO: Love Publishing.

Rothstein, L. F. (1990). *Special education law.* New York: Longman.

Unknown. (1985). *Legal issues in testing.* Clearinghouse on Tests Measurement and Evaluation. Retrieved 10/10/2007 from: http://www.ericdigests.org/pre-927/legal.htm

# Chapter 5

# Legislation Related to the Profession of Speech-Language Pathology

## Introduction

Over the years, several pieces of legislation have affected when, where, and how we deliver our services to individuals who have communication deficits. The purpose of this chapter is to summarize these pieces of legislation.

### Public Laws Enacted by the U.S. Congress with Regard to the Management of Handicapped Individuals (Table 5-1)

**Table 5–1.** An Abbreviated Review of Public Laws Impacting Service Delivery by Speech-Language Pathologists

| Public Law | Year | Description |
|---|---|---|
|  | 1935 | Social Security Act of 1935 |
|  |  | Passed during the Depression, and represented first major entrance of the federal government into the area of health care and health care insurance |

*continues*

**Table 5-1.** *continued*

| Public Law | Year | Description |
|---|---|---|
| | 1935 | Social Security Act of 1935 *continued* <br><br> Basis for Medicare and Medicaid programs <br><br> Provides system of federal benefits for aged persons, blind, dependent and disabled children, maternal and child welfare, public health, and unemployment compensation laws |
| 113 | 1943 | Barden-LaFollette Act <br><br> Made the mentally retarded eligible for vocational rehabilitation services |
| 565 | 1954 | The Rehabilitation Act Amendments of 1954 <br><br> Greatly increased federal funding of rehabilitation including awarding of grants to educational institutions for training of vocational rehabilitation personnel |
| 88-164 | 1963 | Mental Retardation Facilities and Community Health Centers Construction Act of 1963 |
| 333 | 1965 | The Vocational Rehabilitation Amendments of 1965 <br><br> Provided for extended evaluation to determine rehabilitation potential |
| | 1965 | Social Security Act Amendments of 1965 <br><br> Title XVIII: Established Medicare (National Health Insurance for the Aged) <br><br> Part A: Hospital insurance benefits for hospital costs and related posthospital outpatient services <br><br> Part B: Supplemental medical insurance benefits; voluntary; financed by participant with matching funds from general revenues |
| 89-10 | 1965 | The Elementary and Secondary Education Act of 1965 |

**Table 5-1.** *continued*

| Public Law | Year | Description |
|---|---|---|
| 89–313 | 1966 | Federal Assistance to State-Operated and Supported Schools for the Handicapped<br><br>An Amendment to Title I of the Elementary and Secondary Education Act of 1965<br><br>Designed to provide funds for state agencies to better educate handicapped children in state supported and state operated schools |
| 89–750 | 1966 | Elementary and Secondary Education Amendments of 1966.<br><br>Title VI: Education of Handicapped Children<br><br>Section 602: defined "handicapped children" (included hard of hearing, deaf, and special impaired) |
| 91–230 | 1970 | The Education of the Handicapped Act<br><br>An extension of the Elementary and Secondary Act of 1965.<br><br>Authorized funding for development of centers and services, training of special personnel, and research in the education of the handicapped |
| 93–112 | 1973 | The Rehabilitation Act of 1973<br><br>Section 504: To terminate discrimination against handicapped individuals<br><br>Emphasized the rights of all individuals to appropriate services |
| 94–484 | 1973 | The Health Professions Educational Assistance Act of 1973<br><br>Provided funds for grants and contracts in speech-language pathology and audiology |
| 93–380 | 1974 | Education Amendments of 1974<br><br>Section 513: Known as the "Buckley Amendment" or the Family Education Rights and Privacy Act of 1974<br><br>This Act required that states formulate a plan for meeting the needs of all handicapped children |

*continues*

**Table 5-1.** *continued*

| Public Law | Year | Description |
|---|---|---|
| 93–516 | 1974 | The Rehabilitation Act Amendments of 1974<br><br>Clarified the intent of congress to make acts applicable to any person (1) with a mental or physical impairment which affects the person's major life activities and/or (2) for a person who has a record of an impairment or who is regarded as having an impairment. |
| 94–103 | 1974 | The Developmental Disabilities Assistance and Bill of Rights Act |
| 94–142 | 1975 | Education for All Handicapped Children Act of 1975<br><br>All previous legislation led to the development of this Act which authorized congressional funding to provide a "free and appropriate education" for all handicapped children |
| 94–482 | 1976 | The Vocational Education Act Amendments of 1976<br><br>Strengthened the ability of the states to provide increased service to both handicapped children and disabled individuals of all ages who need vocational education |
| 95–207 | 1977 | The Career Education Incentive Act of 1977 |
| 95–156 | 1978 | The Education Amendments of 1978<br><br>Speech-language pathologists may participate in basic skill improvement programming for students whose oral communicative skills are not impaired but could be improved |
| 95–602 | 1978 | The Rehabilitation Services Amendments of 1978<br><br>Comprehensive amendments to provide for rehabilitation services to those handicapped who may never have employment potential, but who can benefit from services to assist them |

**Table 5-1.** *continued*

| Public Law | Year | Description |
|---|---|---|
| 99–457 | 1986 | The Education of the Handicapped Act Amendments of 1986 |
| | | This Act includes provisions for handicapped children of all ages, and "at risk" children between the ages of birth and six, and their families. P.L. 99–457 created a new mandate for state education agencies to serve all 3-, 4-, and 5-year-old children with handicaps by 1990–1991 |
| 101–476 | 1990 | Individuals with Disabilities Education Act |
| | | "Under Part B of IDEA, all eligible preschool and school-aged children and youth with disabilities are entitled to receive a free appropriate public education, including special education and related services" (ASHA, 1990) |
| | 1992 | The Rehabilitation Act of 1973 as Amended by the Rehabilitation Act Amendments of 1992 |
| | | Purpose was to "empower individuals with disabilities to achieve maximum employment, economic self-sufficiency, independence, and inclusion in society" |
| | | Authorized approximately $2 billion dollars in programs and services to provide opportunities for gainful employment and independent living for people with disabilities |
| 101–336 | 1992 | Americans with Disabilities Act |
| | | Civil Rights Bill of the 1990s for people with disabilities |
| 107–110 | 2001 | No Child Left Behind |
| 104–191 | 1996 | Health Insurance Portability and Accountability Act |
| | | Increase protection and efficiency in handling personal health information |

*Note:* Shaded areas are laws that are discussed in this chapter.

## Public Laws Affecting Educational Settings

### Public Law 89-10: The Elementary and Secondary School Act of 1965

The Elementary and Secondary School Act of 1965 (referred to variously in the literature as the Elementary and Secondary Education Act of 1965) (ESEA), was enacted as part of President Lyndon Johnson's War on Poverty as part of his vision of a "Great Society." In 1965, the Equal Opportunity America program funded Head Start in the hope that the provision of cognitive enrichment programs would lead to higher IQs and fewer special education placements for elementary school-age children. Johnson's initiative was based, in part, on President John F. Kennedy's drive to improve the education system in America. In October 1957, when the Russians launched the Sputnik spacecraft (which put them ahead in the "space race"), Kennedy became concerned that the education America's children were receiving was inadequate, particularly in the areas of science and mathematics. After the assassination of President Kennedy in November, 1963, Vice-President Johnson was sworn in as President. President Johnson continued Kennedy's efforts to introduce legislation to improve America's education programs, adding in the need to focus on children from lower socioeconomic backgrounds. As a result of this initiative, the Elementary and Secondary School Act of 1965 was formed to address the need for federal and state funding to compensate schools providing education for the "disadvantaged." Through this program, the legislators were hoping to strengthen and improve educational quality and opportunities in elementary and secondary schools.

It is important to note three facts related to ESEA. First, ESEA was passed on the heels of the Civil Rights Act of 1964, a "landmark anti-discrimination statute." The civil rights activists who lobbied for its passage documented the lack of equality in education of impoverished, minority children. Second, Johnson's bill passed through the congress and was approved in only 87 days. There was very little debate and, consequently, no amendments. It provided funds of $11 billion to public education. Third, since the original enactment of ESEA, it has been reauthorized every five years. The current reauthorization constitutes what is known as the "No Child Left Behind Act of 2001," which is discussed later in this chapter (http://www.answers.com/topic/elementary-and-secondary-education-act; http://en.wikipedia.org/wiki/Elementary_and_Secondary_Education_Act; Vinson, 2007)

## Title I

Money was allocated to the states upon request for local education agencies for the education of children from low-income families. Title I was to provide financial assistance to educational agencies serving areas with concentration of children from low-income families. To qualify as a Title I school, the school's demographics must demonstrate that approximately 40% or more of its students are from low income families (as defined by the United States Census). The primary goal of Title I schools is "to expand and improve their educational programs by various means (including preschool programs) which contribute to meeting the special education needs of educationally deprived children" (Section 201, Elementary and Secondary School Act, 1965). A direct result of Title I was the establishment of Head Start, a program that still operates to prepare low-income and/or handicapped children for success in school. Head Start differed from similar programs that previously had been implemented in that it was holistic in its approach, consisting of four components: education, health, nutrition, and social services (parent education) (Polakow, 1993). Another major difference between this initiative and others with similar goals was that the new programs were justified "in terms of avoidance of future economic costs, rather than on positive humanitarian grounds" (Polakow, 1993, p. 101). It should be mentioned that, even though funding for programming for students with handicaps was possible under Title I, many administrators failed to take advantage of it.

## Title II

Title II of ESEA required that states prepare plans to acquire textbooks and instructional resources needed for this "special" population. Title II authorized allotment of $100 million to states for library resources, textbooks, and other instructional materials.

## Title III

This title encouraged the establishment of additional services and educational centers. These services included guidance counseling, health services, recreation, remedial instruction, and special education programs (although they did not initially consider the handicapped as part of the provisions of Title III.) A later revision of Title III required that 15% of the funding be made available for programs for the handicapped.

## Title IV

Title IV provided funds for educational research and training of educators. It was an amendment to the Cooperative Research Act by authorizing the expenditure of federal dollars to construct national and regional research facilities.

## Title V

This title defined the authority that the Office of Education was to have. It provided funds that were to be used to strengthen state departments of education, and improve or expand a variety of programs and projects designed to improve the effectiveness of operations of state departments of education.

In reality, ESEA (P.L. 89-10) did very little for the education of children with handicaps but, again, its primary focus was to federally mandate the states to upgrade educational facilities for low-income children. However, based on the initiatives put forth in ESEA (1965), laws dedicated to the provision of education services for children with handicaps were enacted. For this reason, I decided that an extended explanation of the history of ESEA was warranted.

## *Public Law 333: Vocational Rehabilitation Amendments of 1965*

The concepts of mainstreaming and least restrictive environment mandate that the personnel required to assist in meeting the needs of children with handicaps in the regular educational settings would be employed. Special services needed to provide appropriate educational programs included speech therapy, social work, occupational therapy, physical therapy, and psychological services. These actions were taken due to underqualified staff and financial problems associated with providing these services for children with handicaps in the public schools.

P.L. 333 expanded services for individuals with handicaps by providing for an extended evaluation to determine rehabilitation potential, including social evaluation, vocational evaluation, psychological evaluation, and medical evaluation. This act enabled Vocational Rehabilitation offices to provide for many handicapped individuals who would have been quickly rejected in previous years.

## *Public Law 89-750: The Elementary and Secondary Education Amendments of 1966*

In 1965, an estimated 5 to 7 million children required some form of special education due to a physical or mental handicap. This led Congress to amend the Elementary and Secondary Education Act of 1965 by creating Title VI, a preliminary effort to provide for publicly funded special education.

The primary provisions of the ESEA of 1966 were as follows:

1. Title VI provided grants for assistance to states for "initiation, expansion and improvement of programs and projects for education of the handicapped at the preschool, elementary, and secondary school levels"
2. Section 602 defined the handicapped child as a child who may be:
   a. mentally retarded
   b. deaf
   c. hearing or speech impaired
   d. emotionally disturbed
   e. visually handicapped
   f. crippled
   g. inflicted by other disabling health problems

States had to submit plans to the Commissioner of Education to receive funding under this amendment. The most important accomplishments of Title VI of P.L. 89-750 were that it provided for the development of the National Advisory Committee on Handicapped Children, and established the Office of Education of the Bureau for the Education and Training of the Handicapped.

## *Public Law 91-230: The Education of the Handicapped Act*

This law was passed by Congress on 04/13/70 as an extension of the Elementary and Secondary Education Act of 1965. It served to repeal Title VI of the Elementary and Secondary Education Act by creating a separate Act, the "Education of the Handicapped Act." This law authorized and provided federal funding grants to states to encourage special education programming. Specifically, the funding grants could be used to:

1. Create services and centers to meet the special needs of the handicapped;
2. Train personnel (including "speech correctionists") to work with handicapped children in educational settings;
3. Fund research in the field of education of the handicapped; and
4. Create special programs for children with specific learning disabilities.

In summary, P.L. 91–230 expressed a moral commitment to children with disabilities and established that those individuals are entitled to the same constitutional rights designated for nondisabled people.

## Public Law 93-380: Education Amendments of 1974 Section 513: Family Education Rights and Privacy Act (FERPA)

The Education Amendments of 1974 was enacted in 1974 when it was signed into law by President Gerald Ford. Actually, they were amendments to P.L. 89–313 (ESEA) that was passed in 1965 to provide funds to better educate children with handicaps in state-supported institutions. Much of the language associated with P.L. 93–380 is affirmed and expanded by P.L. 94–142 with the major emphasis being to set forth procedures and criteria for the making of special grants to state and local educational agencies. It is a federal law, so it only applies to schools that receive federal funding.

### Provisions of Public Law 93-380

There were six provisions of the Education Amendments of 1974:

1. Increasing funding from $100 million to $660 million
2. Requiring states to establish a goal of providing full educational opportunities (mainstreaming) to all children with handicaps as well as educationally deprived children, migratory and delinquent children, and neglected children

3. Establishing procedures to insure that children with handicaps were educated with non-handicapped children, unless stated by the nature or severity of the handicap that mainstreaming would not be satisfactory
4. Stating that procedures used to classify placement of children with handicaps would be administered, but they could not be based on racial or cultural discrimination
5. Providing transportation of children if necessary and beneficial to the student
6. Guaranteeing parental rights (probably the most important provision)

## Section 513: The Buckley Amendment

The Buckley Amendment provided children with handicaps and their parents procedural safeguards in matters concerning identification, evaluation, and educational placement of the child with deficits. In reality, the Buckley Amendment set forth an educational philosophy that recognized the rights of parents and/or students aged 18 years or older to actively be involved in the child's educational process. Parents and students 18 and older could access their educational records and challenge the content (i.e., the accuracy) of the records. In addition, the parents and older students had some degree of control over how the records were disseminated. Thus, the Buckley Amendment deals with access and accuracy of educational records. The Education of All Handicapped Children Act adds the issues of cost and destruction of records.

Part I of the Buckley Amendment states that parents (and students 18 years or over) have the right to "inspect and review all official records, files, and data directly related to their children." Part II states that parents have the right to request a hearing to challenge the presence or absence of pertinent information in the child's educational records. This ensures that all information in the records on their child is accurate and not misleading, and it provides the opportunity for correction or deletion of incorrect or misleading data. If the school does not amend the content specified by the parent and/or eligible student (18 years or older, or enrolled in college), a formal hearing can be held. If there is still no resolution, the parents or eligible student can attach a statement documenting the disagreement over the specific language in the educational record.

Section 438 of the Education Amendments of 1974 declares that parents must give their written permission for the release of confidential information regarding their child.

Section 612 addresses the concept of the "least restrictive environment" (LRE). This section states that the schools must ensure that "to the maximum extent appropriate, handicapped children . . . are educated with children who are not handicapped, and that special classes, separate schooling, or other removal of handicapped children from the regular education environment occurs only when the nature or severity of the handicap is such that education in regular classes with the use of supplementary aids and services cannot be achieved satisfactorily" (Elementary and Secondary Education Amendments of 1974).

Questions about FERPA can be directed to the following address:

Family Policy Compliance Office
U.S. Department of Education
400 Maryland Avenue, SW
Washington, DC 20202-5920

## Public Law 94-142: Education for All Handicapped Children Act (EAHCA) (1975)

EAHCA was passed in 1975 with an implementation date of September 1, 1978. President Gerald Ford was reluctant to sign the bill but did so because there were only seven dissenting votes in congress. The bill authorized the expenditure of federal dollars for special education in order to provide all children with handicaps a free and appropriate education. It mandated public school services for children aged 5 to 21 years, and recommended services for preschoolers aged 3 and 4 years. The primary purpose was to guarantee funding (based on child count) for the implementation of previous legislation. Technically, P.L. 94-142 was an amendment to the Education for the Handicapped Act (P.L. 91-230 of April 13, 1970) that had provided grants to states offering special education. P.L. 94-142 authorized the expenditure of federal funds to subsidize special education provided by the individual states. In reality, it was a funding statute.

Basically, the act was founded on the Constitutional principles of equal protection and due process. The amendment included procedural safeguards, integration, nondiscriminatory testing, and evaluation materials and procedures.

The basic fundamental principles addressed by P.L. 94–142 are:

1. All children with handicaps (who meet eligibility) ages 6 to 18 years must be given education. If the school district serves nonhandicapped students ages 3 to 5 or 19 to 21, then it also must serve the children in those age brackets who are handicapped.
2. The Mainstreaming Mandate means that education must be provided in the least restrictive appropriate placement. This may not necessarily be the best placement. This mandate includes the "separate is not equal" principles from Brown v. the Board of Education.
3. Education is to be individualized and appropriate to the child's unique needs. This is the basis of the individualized education plan (IEP). However, the IEP is not a legally binding contract, and schools are not liable if the goals are not met.
4. The education is to be provided free.
5. "Procedural protections are required to ensure that the substantive requirements are met" (Rothstein, 1990, p. 10). That is to say, due process with regard to identification, evaluation, and placement must be provided.

The major features of P.L. 94–142 are (1) due process, (2) least restrictive environment (placement), (3) nondiscriminatory testing (evaluation), and (4) Child Find (identification). Child Find was implemented in order to get the message to the general public that free and appropriate education services are available in the schools for children with handicaps.

## Special Education and Related Services Defined

EAHCA provided two types of programs: special education and related services. Special education services referred to the primary source of intervention being provided. Children whose primary service is speech-language pathology, and whose speech and/or language deficits are not secondary to other disorders (i.e., hearing impairment, cerebral palsy, Down syndrome, cognitive deficits, etc.) are considered to be enrolled in speech-language therapy as a special education service. "The term 'special education' means specially designed instruction, at no cost to parents, to meet the unique needs of a child with a disability, including (A) instruction conducted in the classroom, in the home, in hospitals and institutions, and in other settings; and (B) instruction in physical education" (EDLAW, Inc., 1997, p. 7)

Related services are those that are provided to a child who is enrolled in a special education classroom placement (whether self-contained or inclusion). For this child, the primary service as designated on his individualized education plan (IEP) is "special education." Related services are

> developmental, corrective, and other supportive services required to assist a handicapped child to benefit from special education and include speech pathology and audiology, psychological services, physical and occupational therapy, recreation, early identification and assessment of disabilities in children, counseling services, and medical services for diagnostic or evaluation purposes. (Rauth, n.d., p. 3)

Related services can include other programs such as transportation, school health services, parent counseling and education, and social work.

The terms "Special education" and "related services" are illustrated in the following two scenarios:

*Scenario 1:* A 9-year-old child, Jason, who has cognitive deficits and is functioning developmentally in the range of 36 to 48 months, is enrolled in a self-contained classroom with children of similar developmental age. As part of his educational program, he receives occupational therapy and speech-language therapy at school. In this scenario, Jason's educational program in the self-contained classroom is his "special education" program. His speech-language therapy and occupational therapy are considered "related services."

*Scenario 2:* Susan, a bright and inquisitive 7-year-old girl, is a student in a "regular" education classroom. She does well academically, interacts with her peers, and adheres to the rules of the classroom. However, Susan has a repaired cleft palate and receives speech-language therapy at school. In this case, the only ancillary service Susan receives is speech therapy; thus, her therapy would be designated as a "special education" service.

### Student Records

One portion of EAHCA was the writing of an individualized education program (IEP) for all children with handicaps in school. The IEP serves as the tool that guarantees the provision of appropriate services for a child who has handicaps. The IEP consisted of seven items:

1. Present levels of educational performance
2. Annual goals
3. Short-term objectives
4. Specific special education and related services to be provided
5. Extent of participation in regular educational programs
6. Projected dates for initiation of services and the anticipated duration of the services
7. Appropriate objective criteria, evaluation procedures and schedules

Three professionals should be at the IEP meeting. The school personnel must document a minimum of three attempts (must include written invitations on standard forms) to have the parent(s) come in and discuss, then sign, the IEP. Once three attempts have been made, the school personnel can implement the IEP without the parents' signatures.

With regard to educational records, there are four major issues:

1. Accuracy: Stigma associated with inaccurate information. This may also affect funding.
2. Access: Protective procedures are needed to prevent unauthorized disclosure of records. State laws regulate access to medical information other than when used for placement decisions.
3. Cost: Reasonable costs may be assessed to parents for copies of records (although this could be up to $1.00 per page, and a record may contain at least 100 pages). Schools must waive this fee if the cost prevents family from obtaining copies of the records.
4. Destruction: State laws differ as to how long records need to be maintained once a student is no longer in the public education system.

## Parent Notification

Notifying parents is absolutely mandatory before preplacement evaluations and initial placement of a child with handicaps in a program providing related services and special education. The EAHCS requires written notice before the agency (1) proposes to initiate or change, or (2) refuses to initiate or change the identification, evaluation, or educational placement of the child or the provision of an appropriate public education placement. Actually, parent notification requirements are in line with the rulings in the Mills v. Board of Education case as part of the due process requirement. (Rothstein, 1990).

## Due Process

The 14th Amendment to the United States Constitution contains equal protection and due process clauses that provide a basis to challenge unequal treatment in the educational process:

> Section 1982 of the Civil Rights Act is the statutory basis through which constitutional and federal statutory violations can be redressed. It provides that individuals deprived of rights, privileges, or immunities of the Constitution or federal laws may bring action in court. (Rothstein, 1990, p. 219)

Complaints under section 504/1983 must be filed within 180 days of the violation. The complaint is filed with the Office of Civil Rights of the Department of Education, and must contain the following:

1. The name, address, and telephone number of the complaining party
2. The basis for the complaint (i.e., handicap discrimination)
3. Who has been affected by the discrimination (may be a group or groups or individual)
4. The name and address of the violating agency
5. The approximate date the violation occurred
6. A brief description of the event
7. The signature of the complaining party (Rothstein, 1990, p. 220).

P.L. 99-372 was passed in 1986 to address the issue of the recovery of attorney's fees incurred during due process procedures.

## Parents' Rights

The "parents' rights" definition as written in P.L. 94-142 has its basis in the Mills v. Board of Education case. Rothstein (1990) writes that:

> The parents in special education situations have important rights and an essential role. Their rights include a right to a hearing and an opportunity to challenge the school's proposed decisions. With that right comes an important role—that of being a participant at almost all stages of the development of an appropriate program and deciding on

an appropriate placement for the child. These rights and roles are not unique to special education. In no other aspect of public education do parents have such an important role and such significant rights. (p. 49)

## Funding

Funding of special education and related services programs in the schools is based on child count. There are some problems with this process, one of which is the complexity of counting handicapped children. The child must fit the definition of handicapped, and also require special education because of the handicap. "The EAHCA defines a handicapped child as one who is mentally retarded, hard of hearing, deaf, speech impaired, visually handicapped, seriously emotionally disturbed, orthopedically impaired, or other health impaired or with specific learning disabilities, who by reason of the handicap requires special education and related services" (Rothstein, 1990, p. 41).

Another problem with the funding is the fact that the funding is based on the average cost of educating a child with handicaps or disabilities. The law does not take into account the wide range of handicaps and disabilities.

## *Public Law 99-457: The Education of the Handicapped Act Amendment of 1986*

### General Information

P.L. 99–457 includes provisions for children of all ages who are handicapped and for children between the ages of birth to 6 years who were "at risk," and for the families of these children. It created a new mandate for state education agencies to serve all 3-, 4-, and 5-year-old children who were handicapped. The mandate had to be met by 1990 to 1991 or the state would lose federal funding. The law has two major portions that are particularly critical to the expansion and improvement of comprehensive services for infants and toddlers and preschoolers:

1. Title I Part H: Program for Infants and Toddlers with Handicaps (birth to age two): Title I (birth to 2) was new and discretionary. These funds could not be used to pay for services that would otherwise be paid for from another source. Also, this tile said that

districts could not reduce the assistance or alter eligibility for Medicaid or Children's Medical Services funds.

2. Title II: Preschool Grants Program (ages 3–5 years): This Title provided incentives for all eligible children with handicaps who would be 3 to 6 years old by the 1990 to 1991 school year. It provides for interagency agreements to share the "free and appropriate education" costs. It also built in penalties for states that did not achieve the full "free and appropriate education" mandate (FAPE) for aged 3–5 children by 1990 to 1991.

3. Title III and IV: Discretionary and Miscellaneous Programs: Programs that provide support to state policy, program development, and implementation could apply for funds from 99 to 457 to offer inservice training for school employees, and to foster research.

As late as 1987, only 28% of children displaying developmental delay were identified prior to school age. Interestingly enough, of the children who were identified, the overwhelming majority was not identified by the medical community. (Rossetti, 1996). This put additional burdens on speech-language pathologists, audiologists, and educators to have adequate assessment instruments to identify developmental disabilities.

Services for children aged birth to two years who were "at risk" or "handicapped" were to be provided. Services for the "at risk" population were discretionary, but if the states provided the service, they had to pay for that programming. For those children who were considered handicapped, services were permissive, but if the state accepted the federal funds, they had to meet all participatory regulations.

There were three purposes of P.L. 99–457. The overriding purpose of P.L. 99–457 was to increase the development of infants who were handicapped by increasing the family's ability to serve their child. The law provided support in order to promote family and child development. The second purpose for serving infants and their families was that it would decrease educational costs of special education programs because the early intervention would minimize the need for special education. Finally, it also was anticipated that this early programming would decrease the likelihood of eventual institutionalization.

## Funding

Funding sources for P.L. 99–457 included all preschool grant funds, all P.L. 94–142 dollars that were generated by children aged 3 to 5 years, and all grants and contracts related to preschool special education funded under the Education of the Handicapped Discretionary Program. Funding was set at $300.00 per year per handicapped child aged 3 to 5 years old.

Funding is different from P.L. 94-142 funding. This funding was based on child count in the schools. P.L. 99-457 funding was different since it was based on the percentage of handicapped children aged birth to two years in the state's total population.

### The Individualized Family Service Plan (IFSP)

Each eligible child must receive a multidisciplinary assessment and have a written IFSP. The IFSP must be reviewed every six months, and rewritten at least annually. The IFSP must include the following:

1. Present levels of development
2. Family strengths and needs
3. Early intervention services needed by the handicapped infant/toddler and family (who, what, where, and frequency of services)
4. Projected dates of services
5. Case manager (from the profession most immediately relevant to the infant/toddler/families' needs and who will be responsible for the implementation of the programs and coordination with other agencies and persons.

### Additional Interpretation

Senate Report 99-315 and House Report 99-860 were developed to assist in the interpretation and implementation of P.L. 99-457.

## Public Law 101-476: Individuals with Disabilities Education Act (IDEA) (1990)

IDEA is an outgrowth of two earlier laws, amending P.L. 94-142 and P.L. 99-457:

1. The Education of All Handicapped Children Act (P.L. 94-142), which was passed in 1975, established funding to provide a free and appropriate public education (FAPE) for all school-aged children with disabilities.

2. P.L. 99-457 was passed in 1986 and extended P.L. 94-142 funding to provide intervention programs for preschool aged children (3-5 years) who had disabilities.

P.L. 101-476 changed the name of the Education of All Handicapped Children Act (EAHCA) to IDEA. Particularly noteworthy is that it changed legislative language to read "individuals with disabilities" instead of "handicapped children." The other major change was the addition of "transition" as a service to be addressed on the individualized education plan (IEP). A requirement is that transition be added to the IEPs by the time the students achieve age 16 years. However, it is strongly encouraged that transition be addressed earlier if appropriate because some children will drop out of school when they turn 16, and some children will require more than two years to meet transition goals due to the severity of their disability.

Part B of IDEA states that all eligible preschoolers and school-aged youth with disabilities are entitled to a free and appropriate education, including special education and related services. Furthermore, the rights of children and youth with disabilities and, and, of their parents are protected by law. It provided assistance in the provision of services and ensures the effectiveness of the program (outcome measures).

Part H or IDEA makes provisions for infants and toddlers, and the parents of these children, to receive educational services. Due to the dependence of infants and toddlers on their parents, the individualized family service plan (IFSP) addresses needs of the families (parents and child). The National Early Childhood Technical Assistance Center (NEC-TAC) prepared guidelines for the IFSP, stating that "respect for family, autonomy, independence, and decision making means that families must be able to choose the level and nature of early intervention's involvement in their life" (NEC-TAC, http://www.nectac.org, n.d.). Families and professionals must operate in concert with each other; this partnership and collaboration are critical in the successful implementation of the IFSP. The IFSP should address the skills the infant or toddler needs to transition to preschool (under Part B). These steps include the following:

1. discussions with, and training of, parents regarding future placements and other matters related to the child's transition;
2. procedures to prepare the child for changes in service delivery, including steps to help the child adjust to, and function in, a new setting;

3. with parental consent, the transmission of information about the child to the local educational agency (NEC-TAC, date unknown).

The IFSP process begins with interaction between a family and the early intervention services agency. Following that, the different disciplines plan and conduct the assessment. The strengths and needs of the child AND the family are noted, and used as the foundation for developing functional outcomes for the child and the family. Then, the IFSP is implemented, and the family and child are formally and informally re-evaluated throughout the process (NEC-TAC, date unknown).

A transition IEP requires all the elements of the IEP as specified in P.L. 94–142, plus the needed transition services. IDEA defines transition services as "a coordinated set of activities for a student, designed with an outcome-oriented" focus. Transition services can refer to skills needed to transition from one level of education to the next (i.e., transition from elementary school to middle school), or from the educational setting to the work force. This may require making a list of the vocational site's responsibilities. The transition IEP must be outcome oriented, and state the desired postschool activities. The set of activities must be based on the needs of the student, and includes needed activities in the areas of:

1. instruction,
2. community experiences,
3. the development of employment and other postschool adult living objectives, and
4. if appropriate, the acquisition of daily living skills and functional vocational evaluation,

that promote movement from school to postschool activities (NAC-TAS).

## No Child Left Behind Act (NCLB)

Passed in 2001, the NCLB heralded a reformation of the American education system by "changing the culture" of schools in America, and by improving student achievement as measured by standardized tests. It is a reauthorization of the Elementary and Secondary Education Act of 1966, a federal law that revamped public education from kindergarten through high school.

NCLB is centered on four themes: (1) accountability for results; (2) an emphasis on doing what works based on scientific research; (3) expanded parental options; and (4) expanded local control and flexibility. ASHA identified five issues that have an impact on the provision of speech-language pathology and audiology in elementary and secondary schools:

1. "highly qualified" teachers and paraprofessionals;
2. use of accommodations, modifications, and alternate assessments for students with disabilities;
3. assessment of English language learners;
4. sanctions for schools identified as in need of improvement, including the provision of supplemental services; and
5. accountability and adequate yearly progress (ASHA, retrieved 10/22/07).

The primary focus of NCLB is school accountability. All students in grades 3 to 8 are to receive annual testing that focuses on reading and mathematics. As required by IDEA, NCLB states that it is a requirement that accommodations for students with disabilities be made.

Appendix 5A is a document from the U.S. Department of Education that defines the terms associated with No Child Left Behind.

## Health Care Legislation Impacting Delivery of SLP Services

Most legislation that relates to health care settings is based on issues related to reimbursement. Other issues of primary concern are those related to liability and malpractice.

### *The Social Security Act of 1935*

This act was passed during the Depression, and represented the first major entrance of the federal government into the area of health care insurance. Eventually, the Social Security Act of 1935 formed the basis for the current Medicaid and Medicare programs. Specifically, the act provides a system of federal benefits for aged persons, blind persons, dependent and disabled children, maternal and child welfare, public health, and unemployment compensation laws.

## Social Security Act Amendments of 1965

Title XVIII of the Social Security Act Amendments of 1965 established Medicare (national health insurance for the aged). Part A provides hospital insurance benefits for hospital costs and related posthospitalization outpatient services.

Part B provides supplemental medical insurance benefits. Part B is a voluntary program. The benefits are financed by the participant with matching funds from general revenues. This program includes physicians' services, lab tests, x-rays, supplies and equipment, and home health care.

Audiology is included under the umbrella of speech-language pathology and is covered under Part A and Part B. The benefits cover nearly everything related to audiology, except for hearing aids and hearing aid evaluations. Also, the participant must have prescription/authorization from a physician for the audiology service to be eligible for Medicare reimbursement.

Title XIX of the Social Security Act Amendments of 1965 initiated Medicaid which established federally supported and state administered programs of health insurance for recipients of public assistance. It also provides benefits to medically indigent persons not on welfare. It is up to individual states as to which services will be provided within the following six categories: inpatient hospital services, outpatient hospital services, laboratory and x-ray services, skilled nursing facility services, physicians' services, and other services as allowed by the state (including speech-language pathology and audiology).

## Social Security Act Amendments of 1972

In 1972, another set of Social Security Act Amendments was passed by the Congress. The 1972 revisions added speech-language pathology services as part of outpatient physical therapy services. Under Part B, speech-language pathologists can get their own provider number if they meet the requirements for designation as a rehabilitation agency.

The 1972 Amendments also established Early and Periodic Screening, Diagnosis, and Treatment Program under Medicaid which provides child health screening (includes speech-language pathology and audiology), hearing aids, and augmentative devices and follow-up treatment for families receiving aid for dependent children.

### Social Security Act Amendments of 1982

The Social Security Act Amendments of 1982 changed reimbursement procedures as a direct result of the Tax Equity and Fiscal Responsibility Act (TEFRA). Previously, hospitals were reimbursed according to actual reported costs of care. Following the 1982 Amendments, hospitals were paid a fixed payment or discharge limit for all hospital-related costs, including speech-language pathology and audiology services. This was done to encourage cost containment.

The 1982 Amendments also added reimbursement for hospice care, including speech-language pathology services for terminally ill patients if services are offered in a manner consistent with accepted standards of practice.

### Social Security Act Amendments of 1983

The Social Security Act Amendments of 1983 reinforced TEFRA by creating PPS (Prospective Payment System). This established reimbursement caps based on a patient's diagnosis or diagnosis-related group (DRG). Arguably, PPS has led to compromises in the quality of care provided by members of medical and allied health professionals.

### Medicare Communication Disorders and Services Act (1984)

The Medicare Communication Disorders and Services Act provided for independent provider status for speech-language pathologists, and coverage for aural rehabilitation services provided by an audiologist. It also permitted the removal of complex eligibility requirements for patients to qualify for audiology services, and provided coverage for individuals who need assistive and augmentative communication devices.

Actually, this Act failed to pass in 1992 and 1993, but in 1994 the technical portions dealing with speech-language pathology and audiology were passed as part of the Social Security Act Amendments of 1994.

## *Medicaid Reform*

Medicaid reform proposals being considered include capping annual growth of federal Medicaid spending at 5 to 7%, which would negatively impact Medicaid and Supplemental Security Income (SSI) recipients. The effort to have a balanced budget by 2002 included caps on several federal entitlement programs including Aid to Families with Dependent Children, SSI, and Medicaid.

It was also necessary to keep an eye on the Individuals with Disabilities Education Act (IDEA) and Americans with Disabilities Act funding in spite of the fact that there are amendments to protect these civil rights statutes.

## *U.S. Public Health Service Act (1944)*

The U.S. Public Health Service Act (1944) was passed for the sole purpose of consolidating all legislation relating to national public health services. Subsequent amendments affecting speech-language pathologists are as follows:

### Title XIII: Health Maintenance Organization Act of 1973

This Act creates the provision of basic medical services under a fixed periodic payment community rating system, including physician services, inpatient and outpatient services, medically necessary emergency health services, short-term outpatient evaluation services, and crisis intervention mental health services (limited to 20 visits).

In addition, patients can contract for supplemental health services, including intermediate and long-term care, vision care, dental and mental health services, and prescription drugs.

With regard to authorization for medical services, the Federal HMO Act of 1973 reads as follows:

> Federally qualified HMOs must provide or arrange for outpatient service and inpatient hospital services which shall include short-term rehabilitation and physical therapy, the provision of which the HMO determines can be expected to result in the significant improvement of a member's condition within a period of two months. (Code of Federal Regulations, Title 42, Section 110102 [1990])

Unfortunately, the period of two months is most frequently interpreted as a maximum of two months, instead of a minimum of two months as was the intention of the act (Frattali, 1999).

### The Social Security Act Amendments of 1976

The Social Security Act Amendments in 1976 were less stringent than those of previous years. If the health maintenance organization (HMO) is receiving Medicare/Medicaid reimbursement, it must be federally qualified. These amendments also limited speech-language pathology and audiology services by saying that the HMO can determine the conditions under which improvement is expected in two months.

### Technology-Related Assistance for Individuals with Disabilities Act of 1988

This act was passed to increase availability and funding for assistive technology.

### Numerous Omnibus Budget Reconciliation Acts

The Omnibus Budget Reconciliation Acts were developed to instruct authorizing committees to cut spending in health programs.

The years 1980, 1985, 1986, 1989, and 1990 are significant for speech-language pathology and/or audiology because they contained provisions that related directly to the delivery of speech-language pathology and audiology services. The 1980 act, which became effective on January 1, 1981, enabled speech-language pathologists to write their own treatment plans for Medicare beneficiaries. In 1987, the act increased access to speech-language pathology services for residents of nursing homes.

## *Public Law 101–518: Section 4206 (Patient Self-Determination Act of 1990)*

Section 4206 of Public Law 101–518 states that "all Medicare and Medicaid provider organizations such as hospitals, nursing homes, and home health agencies must: (a) provide information to patients regarding the right to refuse medical treatment and to formulate advance directives, (b) maintain documentation and records of advance directives, (c) review advance directives periodically, (d) comply with directives as dictated by state law, and (e) educate staff and the community on issues concerning advance directives" (Sabatino & Gottlich, 1991). According to Sabatino and Gottlich, the primary goals of the Patient Self-Determination Act were to encourage patient autonomy and to give patients the right to execute advance directives. In addition, the act sought to "eliminate problems associated with terminating life sustaining treatment for incompetent patients by mandating increased communication about patients' rights between patients and their health care providers" (Mulholland, 1991, p. 616).

Applebaum and Grisso (1998) put forth four categories of legal standards that should be taken into consideration and evaluated when determining an individual's competence:

1. Ability to communicate choices consistently;
2. Ability to understand relevant information about a treatment decision;
3. Ability to comprehend a situation and its probable consequences; and
4. Ability to use logical reasoning to compare benefits and risks of treatment options.

They further maintain that competent patients should have the right to refuse any type of treatment, regardless of the consequences. In addition, the court ruled that incompetent patients lose the right to refuse treatment, and decisions are made for them (Landes, 1999).

## Public Laws Affecting Employment of Persons with Disabilities

### *Americans with Disabilities Act (Public Law 101-336)*

The Americans with Disabilities Act is considered to be the Civil Rights bill of the 1990s for people with disabilities. Passed by Congress in 1990 and signed into law by President George H. W. Bush, the ADA took effect on July 26, 1992. ADA prohibits discrimination on the basis of disability in (1) private sector employment (Title I), (2) services rendered by state and local governments (Title II), (3) places of public accommodation (Title III), (4) transportation (Title IV), and (5) telecommunication services (Title V).

The U.S. Equal Employment Opportunity Commission (EEOC) defines an individual with a disability as "a person who:

1. Has a physical or mental impairment that substantially limits one or more major life activities
2. Has a record of such an impairment; or
3. Is regarded as having such an impairment" (EEOC, 2007, p. 1).

An employer must make accommodations for an employee who is disabled, but the individual must be able, with or without "reasonable accommodations" to perform the duties of the job. EEOC (1990) defines reasonable accommodations as follows: "Reasonable accommodation may include, but is not limited to:

1. making existing facilities used by employees readily accessible to and usable by persons with disabilities;
2. job restructuring, modifying work schedules, reassignment to a vacant position;
3. acquiring or modifying equipment or devices, adjusting modifying examinations, training materials, or policies, and providing qualified readers or interpreters" (p. 1).

An employer is not expected to make accommodations for an employee if it creates "undue hardship" on the employer. "Undue hardship is defined as an action requiring significant difficulty or expense when considered in light of factors such as an employer's size, financial resources and the nature and structure of its operation" (EEOC, 1990, p. 1).

ADA is based on The Rehabilitation Act of 1973 as amended by the Rehabilitation Act Amendments of 1992. The purpose is to empower individuals who have disabilities to achieve in four areas: employment, economic self-sufficiency, personal independence, and inclusion in the general population. To achieve this goal, ADA ensures coordination and interagency cooperation in implementing the Rehabilitation Act of 1973, its amendments in 1992, and ADA.

## Title I: Employment

"Covered entity" refers "to an employment agency, labor organization, or joint labor-management committee, and is generally an employer engaged in interstate commerce and having 15 or more workers." (Elementary and Secondary Education Act, October. 2007). According to ADA, a covered entity cannot discriminate against an employee who has a disability, but is qualified to do the job. "Discrimination, among other things, may include limiting or classifying a job applicant or employee in an adverse way, denying employment opportunities to people who truly qualify, or not making reasonable accommodations to the known physical or mental limitations of disabled employees, not advancing employees with disabilities in the business, and/or not providing needed accommodations in training" (Elementary and Secondary Education Act, 2007).

## Title II: Public Services (and Public Transporation)

Section I of Title II comprises public agencies and requires them to "comply with regulations similar to Section 504 of the Rehabilitation Act." These agencies (local, county, state, federal governments and their units) must comply with access standards for all programs they offer. This can refer to physical access and "access that might be obstructed by discriminatory policies or procedures of the entity" (Elementary and Secondary Education Act, 2007).

Section II of Title II specifically addresses access to public transportation. This includes planes, trains, and buses.

> Both sections state that no qualified individual with a disability shall be subjected to discrimination or excluded from the benefits of the services, programs, or activities of a public entity, or be subjected to discrimination by any such entity due to his or her disability. (Elementary and Secondary Education Act, 2007)

## Title III: Public Accommodations (and Commercial Facilities)

Public accommodations "include most places of lodging (such as inns and hotels), recreation, transportation, education, and dining, along with stores, care providers, and places of public displays, among other things" (Elementary and Secondary Education Act, 2007). Persons with disabilities should be able to equally enjoy and participate in the programs, facilities, services, and goods of any *public* place. Certain private organizations and religions entities are not bound by Title III.

## Title IV: Communications

This is an amendment of the 1934 Communications Act. It is estimated that there are approximately 1600 telecommunication companies in the United States. They must "take steps to ensure functionally equivalent services for consumers with disabilities, notably those who are deaf or hard of hearing and those with speech impairments" (Elementary and Secondary Education Act, 2007).

## Title V: Miscellaneous Provisions

This includes all technical provisions and states that ADA cannot "amend, override, or cancel anything in Section 504 (discussed earlier in this chapter).

Additional information on ADA is available in a booklet entitled, "The Americans with Disabilities Act: Questions and Answers" and is available from the US. Equal Employment Opportunity Commission (1801 L Street NW, Washington, DC 20507).

## Technology-Related Assistance for Individuals with Disabilities Act Amendments of 1994 (Tech Act)

Public Law 103-218 (1988) is "a federal competitive grants program which provides monies for states to establish a statewide, consumer-responsive service delivery system designed to effect systems change regarding assistive technology" (Ourand & Gray, 1997, p. 345). The original act delineated a broad definition of assistive technology that encompasses all devices regardless of the level of technology.

The programs under the Tech Act do not necessarily provide direct funding for AAC services and devices. Rather, "most states use Tech Act grants to fund broad programs to disseminate information and provide referrals to increase access to assistive technology" (Ourand & Gray, 1997, p. 345).

## Health Insurance Portability and Accountability Act (HIPAA)

In 1996, the United States Congress enacted the Health Insurance Portability and Accountability Act (P.L. 104-191), commonly referred to as HIPAA. HIPAA consists of three regulations: (1) privacy of protected health information; (2) transactions associated with electronic data interchange, and (3) security of protected health information (PHI). One purpose of the original law was to protect employees' insurance coverage when they change, or lose, their job. Over time, the larger emphasis became privacy of health information about patients. In addition, it was developed to establish national standards for electronic health care transactions and code sets. The ultimate goal was to increase efficiency in health care arenas by promoting electronic interchange of data in the health professions and by eliminating paper forms (Phoenix Health Systems, 2005). Not only is patients' information protected; there is also a financial side to the law. It is estimated that the implementation of HIPAA will result in a $29.9 billion dollar savings for the health care industry over the first 10 years of implementation. The Health Information Privacy component of the law, "among other things, allows for more consumer control over health information, sets boundaries on medical record use and release, provides safeguards to ensure security of personal health information, and provides for accountability for medical records use and release" (ASHA, 2002a).

The major focus of HIPAA is the "Privacy Rule" component. The Privacy Rule provides specifics on how patients' PHI can be used and disclosed. It also provides standards that enable patients to comprehend and control how their personal health information is used.

> A major goal of the Privacy Rule is to assure that individuals' health information is properly protected while allowing the flow of health information needed to provide and promote high quality health care and to protect the public's health and well being. The Rule strikes a balance that permits important uses of information, while protecting the privacy of people who seek care and healing. Given that the health care marketplace is diverse, the Rule is designed to be flexible and comprehensive to cover the variety of uses and disclosures that need to be addressed. (Office for Civil Rights, 2003, p. 1)

In addition to the Privacy Rule, there are Administrative Simplification Rules (Title II) that are composed of Sections 261–264 of HIPAA. The purpose of the Administrative Simplification Rules is to provide standards governing electronic exchange of health information, insuring that privacy and security of PHI are maintained. The benefits that HIPAA holds for patients includes decreasing administrative costs, increasing the efficiency in handling PHI, protecting health information, enhancing security for electronic health transactions, and complying with federal laws (Unpublished document, James Madison University, n.d.). Basically, the goal was to establish a single, standard format for electronic submissions. This section of the law calls for the development of electronic transaction code sets for electronic data interchange (EDI). It was mandated that all health care providers "will be able to use this electronic format to bill their services and all health plans will be required to accept the standard electronic claims, referral authorizations, and other transactions" (ASHA, 2002a). Standards for the security of individual health information and electronic signature use were established. These standards require protection of health care information that is electronically collected, maintained, utilized, or transmitted. It also applies these standards to the storage of patient files. These files must be in a protected area and/or under lock and key.

Rules also were developed regarding "business associates." "In general, a business associate is a person or organization, other than a member of a covered entity's workforce, that performs certain functions or activities on behalf of, or provides services to, a covered entity that involve the use or disclosure of individually identifiable health information. Business associate functions or activities on behalf of a covered entity include claims processing, data analysis, utilization review, and billing" (Office of Civil Rights, 2003, p. 3). A contract must be developed between a covered entity and a business associate to ensure the privacy and proper disclosure of PHI. Safeguards and procedures that define use of the PHI and prevent any violations of the Privacy Rule should be documented.

Covered entities can disclose PHI for purposes of treatment, payment, and/or health care operations (TPO). The law defines treatment as "the provision, coordination, or management of health care and related services for an individual by one or more health care providers, including consultation between providers regarding a patient and referral of a patient by one provider to another" (OCR, 2003, p. 5). Payment refers to such activities as obtaining "premiums, determine or fulfill responsibilities for coverage and provision of benefits, and furnish or obtain reimbursement for health care delivered to an individuals and activities of a health care provider to obtain payment or be reimbursed for the provision of health care to an individual" (OCR, 2003, p. 5).

The final segment of TPO, Health Care Operations, is defined by the Office of Civil Rights (2003) as any of the following:

(a) quality assessment and improvement activities, including case management and care coordination; (b) competency assurance activities, including provider or health plan performance evaluation, credentialing, and accreditation; (c) conducting or arranging for medical reviews, audits, or legal services, including fraud and abuse detection and compliance programs; (d) specified insurance functions, such as underwriting, risk rating, and reinsuring risk; (e) business planning, development, management, and administration; and (f) business management and general administrative activities of the entity, including but not limited to : de-identifying protected health information, creating a limited data set, and certain fundraising for the benefit of the covered entity. (p. 5)

Regardless of the reason(s) for the disclosure, OCR has adopted a "minimum necessary" stance on the release of PHI. This means that the covered entity will take care to release only the absolutely necessary PHI.

A basic plan for implementing HIPAA is as follows:

1. Train all employees on the law and associated policies and procedures.
2. Conduct a "gap analysis" to determine where PHI could be disclosed improperly, then address those instances.
3. Provide a notice of privacy practices to each patient, and have him or her sign acknowledging receipt of the privacy practices of that particular entity
4. Obtain consent from the patient to use and disclose PHI from treatment, payment, and health care operations;
5. Obtain consent from the patient to use PHI for nonhealth purposes.
6. Develop advance notice of the provider's policies with regard to disclosure.
7. Inform the patient that he/she has the right to see and correct health records and obtain disclosure history.
8. Obtain the patient's signature on a release of medical information (for billing or for treatment).
9. Meet with each patient to explain the rules of HIPAA and what your office is doing to comply with the standards set forth in the act. Each agency is responsible for providing a detailed written plan of its health information practices, and the patient must sign that he/she has been given a copy of this policy.
10. If patient information is transmitted electronically as in an E-mail, the information should be encrypted.
11. Establish policies and procedures:
    a. Who has the authority to release PHI?
    b. Designate a responsible staff member to oversee and regulate the use of PHI.
    c. Develop a records management system that complies with the terms of HIPAA
    d. Establish fax policies and develop a new cover sheet indicating that any disclosure of PHI in the fax has been done in compliance with HIPAA.

e. Develop and place policies and procedures in a handbook that is available for review by all staff members and student trainees.

f. Shred all patient-related documents when they are no longer needed.

The HIPAA Security Rule addresses privacy issues related to electronic protected health information, referred to as EPHI. With regard to developing policies and procedures, it is suggested that the following issues be addressed:

1. "to ensure the confidentiality, integrity, and availability of all EPHI;
2. "to protect against reasonable anticipated threats or hazards to the security of integrity of EPHI;
3. "and to prohibit uses and disclosures not permitted or required under the privacy rule" (Cornett, 2007, p. 289).
4. analysis of risk factors that could result in inadvertent disclosure of EPHI
5. policies and procedures to be followed in the event of intentional and/or inadvertent disclosure of EPHI
6. physical safeguards: "facility access, validation procedures, and standards for devices and media controls" (Cornett, p. 289)
7. technical safeguards: "ensure access control on systems that maintain EPHI, security of EPHI transmissions, audit controls, and authentication procedures" (Cornett, p. 289).

The term "covered entity" was devised to identify organizations that need to be in compliance with the HIPAA. These organizations include health care providers, health care clearinghouses, and health plans. Health care providers are listed as including "individual physicians, physician group practices, dentists, hospitals, nursing facilities, other health care practitioners (such as speech-language pathologists, audiologists, physical therapists, occupational therapists, etc.). So, "any health care provider or insurance entity that maintains or transmits 'individually identifiable health information,' referred to as 'protected information' about a patient or client is deemed a 'covered entity'" (ASHA, 2002). Furthermore, any agencies with which PHI is shared about a patient, such as a hearing aid marketer, would be identified as a "business associate" and would be subject to the regulations associated with HIPAA.

### Noncompliance

Individuals or agencies that fail to comply with the rules and regulations of HIPAA are subject to penalties, primarily financial, that would be imposed by the Office of Civil Rights in the Health and Human Services Office. Civil penalties ranging from $100.00 per violation and a maximum of $25,000.00 per year can be imposed. If it is determined that the violations are malicious and result in personal gain (for example, selling PHI), criminal penalties would be implemented. These include penalties ranging from one year in prison and a $50,000 fine up to 10 years in prison and a financial penalty up to $250,000.00. (ASHA, 2002b, Rao, 2007)

Table 5-2 sums up the terms related to the HIPAA Privacy Rule.

### National Provider Identifier

Every practitioner involved in delivery of health care services must obtain a National Provider Identifier (NPI). This can be done by going to the NPI Web site (https://nppes.cms.hhs.gov), or contacting the NPI Enumerator at P.O. Box 6059/Fargo, ND 58108-6059. The toll-free telephone number is 1-800-465-3203. The NPI is noted on every piece of health care documentation related to patient care.

**Table 5–2.** Terms Related to the HIPAA Privacy Rule

**Covered entity:** a health plan, health care clearinghouse, or health care provider that transmits any health information in electronic form in connection with a standard financial or administrative transaction listed in Section 1173(1)(1) of the act and Section 160.103 of the final rule.

**Designated record set:** a group of records maintained by or for a covered entity, including the medical records and billing records about individuals maintained by or for a covered health care provider; the enrollment, payment, claims, adjudication, and case for medical management record systems maintained by or for a health plan; or data used, in whole or in part, by or for the covered entity to make decisions about individuals.

**Table 5–2.** *continued*

**Disclosure:** release, transfer, provision of access to, or divulging in any other manner of information outside the entity holding the information

**Health information:** any information, whether oral or recorded in any form or medium, that is created or received by a health care provider, health plan, public health authority, employer, life insurer, school or university, or health care clearinghouse, that relates to the past, present, or future physical or mental health or condition of an individual, the provision of health care to the individual, or the past, present, or future payment for the provision of health care to the individual.

**Individually identifiable health information:** a subset of health information, including demographic information collected from an individual, that is created or received by a health care provider, health plan, employer, or health care clearinghouse and that relates to the past, present, or future physical or mental health or condition of an individual; the provision of health care to an individual; or the past, present, or future payment for the provision of health care to an individual. There must be a reasonable basis to believe the information can be used to identify the individual.

**Protected health information:** individually identifiable health information that is transmitted by electronic media; maintained in any medium described in the definition of electronic media; or transmitted or maintained in any other form or medium. Protected health information excludes individually identifiable health information in education records covered by the Family Educational Right and Privacy Act, as amended, 20 U.S.C. 1232g, and Records described at 20 U.S.C. 1232g(a)(4)(B)(iv).

**Use:** with respect to individually identifiable health information, the sharing, employment, application, examination, or analysis of such information within an entity that maintains such information.

*Source:* From "Service Delivery in Health Care Settings" by B. S. Cornett, in *Professional Issues in Speech-Language Pathology and Audiology* (3rd ed., p. 289) by R. Lubinski, L. C. Golper, and C. M. Frattali (Eds.). Copyright 2007 by Thomson Delmar Learning, 2007. Reprinted with permission.

## Summary

The intent of this chapter was to summarize the passages of numerous pieces of legislation that can impact our service delivery in all settings. Funding for seeing patients often hinges on compliance with these laws. Clinicians are encouraged to be familiar with the laws, and keep up with current legislation (the ASHA Leader keeps us well-informed) that affects the profession of speech-language pathology.

## References

American Speech-Language-Hearing Association. (2002a). *Legislative issues: Health Insurance Portability and Accountability Act—Gateway to Implementation.* Rockville, MD: Author.

American Speech-Language-Hearing Association. (2002b). *Legislative issues: HIPAA: General Information.* Rockville, MD: Author.

Applebaum, P. S., & Grisso, T. (1988). Assessing patients' capacities to consent to treatment. *New England Journal of Medicine, 319,* 1635–2638.

Ballard, J., Ramirez, B. A., & Weintraub, F. J. (1982). *Special education in America: Its legal and governmental foundations.* Reston, VA: Council for Exceptional Children.

Cornett, B. S. (2007). Service delivery in health care settings. In R. Lubinski, L. C. Golper, & C. M. Frattali (Eds.), *Professional issues in speech-language pathology and audiology* (3rd ed.). Clifton Park, NY: Thomson Delmar Learning.

Digest of Public General Bills and Resolutions. (1974). 93/2, Library of Congress, Part 1.

EDLAW, Inc. (1997). *Individuals with Disabilities Education Act.* Hollywood, FL: Author.

Elementary and Secondary Education Act. (n.d.) *Answers.com.* Retrieved March 3, 2009, from http://www.answers.com/topic/elementary-and-secondary-education-act

Elementary and Secondary Education Act. (2007). In *Wikipedia, the Free Encyclopedia.* Retrieved March 3, 2009, from http://en.wikipedia.org/wiki/Elementary_and_Secondary_Education_Act

Elementary and Secondary Education Amendments of 1974. 93/2, Report No. 93-805.

Frattali, C. M. (1999). Measuring and managing outcomes. In B. S. Cornett, *Clinical practice management for speech-language pathologists* (pp. 29–52). Gaithersburg, MD: Aspen.

Gottlich V. (1990).The effects of the Cruzan case on the rights of elderly clients. *Clearinghouse Review, 24*, 663–670.

Landes, T. L. (1999). Ethical issues involved in patients' rights to refuse artificially administered nutrition and hydration and implications for the speech-language pathologist. *American Journal of Speech-Language Pathology, 8(2)*.

Mulholland, K. C. (1991). Protecting the right to die: The patient self-determination act of 1990. *Harvard Journal on Legislation, 28*, 609–630.

NEC-TAC. (n.d.). http://www.nectac.org

Office for Civil Rights. (2003). *Summary of the HIPAA Privacy Rule.* Washington, DC: United States Department of Health and Human Services.

Ourand, P. R., & Gray, S. (1997). Funding and legal issues in augmentative and alternative communication. In S. L. Glennen & D. C. DeCoste (Eds.), *Handbook of augmentative and alternative communication* (pp. 335–360). San Diego, CA: Singular.

Personal communication of unpublished document. (n.d.). James Madison University.

Phoenix Health Systems. (2005, July). *HIPAA Primer.* Retrieved June 2005, from: http://www.hipaadvisory.com/REGS/HIPAApimer.htm

Polakow, V. (1993). *Lives on the edge: Single mothers and their children in the other America.* Chicago: University of Chicago Press.

Rao, P. (2007). Policies and procedures. In R. Lubinski, L. C. Golper, & C. M. Frattali (Eds.), *Professional issues in speech-language pathology and audiology* (3rd ed., pp. 411–429). Clifton Park, NY: Thomson Delmar Learning.

Rauth, M. (n.d.). *A guide to understanding the Education for All Handicapped Children Act (P.L. 94-142).* Washington, DC: American Federation of Teachers, AFL-CIO.

Rossetti, L. (1986). *High-risk infants: Identification, assessment, and intervention.* Boston: College-Hill Press.

Rothstein, L. (1990). *Special Education Law.* New York: Longman.

Sabatino, C. P., & Gottlich, V. (1991). Seeking self-determination in the Patient Self-Determination Act. *Clearinghouse Review, 25*, 639–647.

United States Department of Health and Human Services. (2007). *Protecting the privacy of patients' health information.* Washington, DC: Author.

U.S. Department of Education. (2007). Retrieved October 22, 2007, from www.education.com/reference/article/Ref_Glossary_Terms

U.S. Equal Employment Opportunity Commission. (1997). *Facts about the Americans with Disabilities Act.* Retrieved October, 2007, from http://www.eeoc.gov/facts/fs-ada.html

Vinson, B. P. (2007). *Language disorders across the lifespan* (2nd ed.). Clifton Park, NY: Thomson Delmar Learning.

## APPENDIX 5A
## Glossary of Terms: No Child Left Behind*

**Accountability System:** Each state sets academic standards for what every child should know and learn. Student academic achievement is measured for every child, every year. The results of these annual tests are reported to the public.

**Achievement Gap:** The difference between how well low-income and minority children perform on standardized tests as compared with their peers. For many years, low-income and minority children have been falling behind their white peers in terms of academic achievement.

**Adequate Yearly Progress (AYP):** An individual state's measure of yearly progress toward achieving state academic standards. "Adequate Yearly Progress" is the minimum level of improvement that states, school districts and schools musts achieve each year.

**Alternative Certification:** Most teachers are required to have both a college degree in education and a state certification before they can enter the classroom. *No Child Left Behind* encourages states to offer other methods of qualification that allow talented individuals to teach subjects they know.

**Assessment:** Another word for "test." Under *No Child Left Behind*, tests are aligned with academic standards. Beginning in the 2002 to 2003 school year, schools must administer tests in each of three grade spans: grades 3 to 5, grades 6 to 9, and grades 10 to 12 in all schools. Beginning in 2005–2006 school year, tests must be administered every year in grades 3 through 8 in math and reading. Beginning in the 2007–2008 school year, science achievement must also be tested.

**Charter School:** Charter schools are independent public schools designed and operated by educators, parents, community leaders, educational entrepreneurs, and others. They are sponsored by designated local or state educational organizations, which monitor their quality and effectiveness but allow them to operate outside of the traditional system of public schools.

**Comprehensive Corrective Action:** The ability to understand and gain meaning from what has been read. When a school or school district does not make yearly progress, the state will place it under a "Corrective Action Plan." The plan will include resources to improve teaching, administration, or curriculum. If a school continues to be identified as in need of improvement, then the state has increased authority to make any necessary, additional changes to ensure improvement.

**Disaggregated Data:** "Disaggregate" means to separate a whole into its parts. In education, this term means that test results are sorted into groups of students who are economically disadvantaged, from racial and ethnic minority groups, have disabilities, or have limited English fluency. This practice allows parents and teachers to see more than just the average score for their child's school. Instead, parents and teachers can see how each student group is performing.

**Distinguished Schools:** Awards granted to schools when they make major gains in achievement.

**Early Reading First:** A nationwide effort to provide funds to school districts and other public or private organizations that serve children from low-income families. The Department of Education will make competitive 6-year grants to local education agencies to support early language, literacy, and prereading development of preschool-age children, particularly those from low-income families.

**Elementary and Secondary Education Act (ESEA):** ESEA, which was first enacted in 1965, is the principle federal law affecting K to 12 education. The *No Child Left Behind* Act is the most recent reauthorization of the ESEA.

**Flexibility:** Refers to a new way of funding public education. The *No Child Left Behind* Act gives states and school districts unprecedented authority in the use of federal education dollars in exchange for strong accountability for results.

**Fluency:** The capacity to read text accurately and quickly.

**Local Education Agency:** (LEA) is a public board of education or other public authority within a State, which maintains administrative control of public elementary or secondary schools in a city, county, township, school district, or other political subdivision of a state.

**National Assessment of Educational Progress:** An independent benchmark, NAEP is the only nationally representative and continuing assessment of what American students know and can do in various subject areas. Since 1969, The National Center for Education Statistics has conducted NAEP assessments in reading, mathematics, science, writing, U.S. history, geography, civics, and the arts.

**Phonemic Awareness:** The ability to hear and identify individual sounds—or phonemes—in spoken words.

**Phonics:** The relationship between the letters of written language and the sounds of spoken language.

**Public School Choice:** Students in schools identified as in need of improvement will have the option to transfer to better public schools in their districts. The school districts will be required to provide transportation to the students. Priority will be givn to low-income students.

**Reading First:** A bold new national initiative aimed at helping every child in every state become a successful reader.

**State Educational Agency:** (SEA) is the agency primarily responsible for the State supervision of public elementary and secondary schools.

**Supplemental Services:** Students from low-income families who are attending schools that have been identified as in need of improvement for two years will be eligible to receive outside tutoring or academic assistance. Parents can choose the appropriate services for their child from a list of approved providers. The school district will purchase the services.

**Teacher Quality:** To ensure that every classroom has a highly qualified teacher, states and districts around the country are using innovative programs to address immediate and long-term needs, including alternative recruitment strategies, new approaches to professional development, financial incentive programs, partnerships with local universities, and much more.

**Title I:** The first section of the ESEA, Title I refers to programs aimed at America's most disadvantaged students. Title I Part A provides assistance to improve the teaching and learning of children in high-poverty schools to enable those children to meet challenging State academic content and performance standards. Title I reaches about 12.5 million students enrolled in both public and private schools.

**Transferability:** A new ESEA flexibility authority that allows states and local educational agencies (LEAs) to transfer a portion of the funds that they receive under certain Federal programs to other programs that most effectively address their unique needs to certain activities under Title I.

**Unsafe School Choice Option:** Student who attend persistently dangerous public schools or have been victims of violent crime at school are allowed to transfer to a safer public school.

**Vocabulary:** The words students must know to read effectively.

---

*Source: U.S. Department of Education, released July 26, 2007.

*Chapter 6*

# Ethics in Speech-Language Pathology

## What Is Ethics?

Several components must be considered when trying to define ethics. These are listed below and defined:

1. Morals: Conduct or behavior that is judged to be "good or bad."
2. Values: Whatever is deemed proper, desirable, or worthwhile.
3. Ethics: The science or philosophy of balancing values.
4. Law: Rules of conduct that are derived from cultural or community standards of moral and ethical behavior.
5. Clinical Ethics: The identification, analysis, and resolution of moral problems concerning a particular patient.
6. Professional Ethics: The standards or rules of professional behavior which are set out by a profession. Often these rules are detailed in a Code of Ethics. Professional behavior issues include: billing for services not rendered, licensure, malpractice, conflict of interest.
7. Paternalism: The practice of overriding or ignoring a person's preferences in order to benefit them or enhance their welfare (Sharp, 1998).

Ethics can be difficult to define! In his book, *Professional Ethics for Audiologists and Speech-Language Pathologists*, David Resnick (1993) offers 10 definitions of "ethics" in the preface and beginning of Chapter 1:

> "In general, the practice of human conduct according to certain specified principles" (i.e., the ASHA Code of Ethics) (p. xvi)

> "On an individual level, mans' behaving in ways that demonstrate genuine concern for the well-being of people without the motivation of self-interest" (p. xvii)

> "The study of standards of conduct and moral judgment; the system or code of morals of a particular person, religion, group, profession, and so forth" (p. 2)

> "A system of conduct that is painstakingly developed to guide the practice of a specific discipline" (p. 2)

> "The study of human conduct in light of specified moral principles . . . ethical action is behavior consistent with society's security, order, and growth" (p. 2)

> "Obedience to the principles and rules of conduct for an entire profession" (p. 4)

> "A system of disciplined reflection on moral intuitions and moral choices. Ethics attempts to compare beliefs and intuitions and draw inferences to develop rules of conduct about them and to articulate principles that might underlie the rules" (p. 9)

> "What we mean when we say something is right or wrong" (p. 9)

> The integration of "rules and principles with knowledge of facts relevant to a particular sphere of life such as medicine, psychology, audiology, speech-language pathology, or even the total job environment" (p. 9)

> "Allows great emphasis to be placed on the giving of a service to humankind without the need for self-interest" (p. 9)

In Lubinski and Frattali's book, *Professional Issues in Speech-Language Pathology and Audiology* (1994), Charlena Seymour wrote or quoted six definitions on one page. These included the following:

"Simply doing the right thing according to accepted standards of our specific community, culture, or profession" (p. 62)

"Part of philosophy and uses reason, logic, concepts and philosophical explanations to analyze its problems and find answers" (p. 62)

"A moral philosophy that examines the truths and principles of conduct in a systematic way" (p. 62)

"The part of philosophy that is concerned with living well, being a good person, doing the right thing, and wanting the right things in life" (Solomon, 1984)

"Ethics refers both to a discipline—the study of our values and their justification and to the subject matter of that discipline— the actual values and rules of conduct by which we live" (Solomon, 1984) (in Seymour, 1994, p. 62)

Harris (1986, p. 2): "1. the study of standards of conduct and moral judgment; moral philosophy 2. a treatise on this study; book about morals. 3. the system or code of morals of a particular philosopher, religion, group, profession" (p. 62).

## Why Are There More Ethical Dilemmas in the Current Two Decades Than Previously?

One reason for the increase in ethical dilemmas is the tremendous advances in medical technology that increase the ability of the medical profession to keep people alive longer than in the past. For example, premature and very low birth weight babies are surviving and, frequently, are children who have special needs when they become eligible for public school services. Thus, speech-language pathologists in the schools are seeing more complicated and medically compromised children than at any time in the past.

Another concern is that there is a growing distrust of the medical profession. Via Internet connections, patients can find out if there are sanctions against their chosen physicians and clinicians, as well as if he or she has had malpractice suits filed. Also, one hears more often in the news about the inadequate preparation of physicians, and about their prescribing medications that are eventually proven to be more harmful than good. Although this is a problem that originates with the pharmaceutical companies, the physician may take the brunt of the patient's angst because he or she prescribed the medication.

Another situation that enhances the possibility of ethical dilemmas is that there is increasing participation of patients in their own health care. They ask more questions, they often are more informed than patients in the past, and they may challenge their physician's decisions. This type of interaction may put the physician into a situation with which he may not feel professionally comfortable, but has an obligation and desire to hear what the patient thinks, and then come up with a compromised decision. Patients have more rights in this century than they did in the previous one. The physician must balance the patient's wishes and rights with his or her own medical expertise. For example, some patients may request to be dismissed from the hospital, which may be in conflict with the physician's advice.

There are three ethical situations specific to the school-based speech-language pathologist. One dilemma involves the denial of services to children who need assistance, yet due to stringent eligibility criteria (which is sometimes implemented to keep caseloads at a reasonable level), the children do not qualify for services. A second issue is that of serving severely involved children in large groups. One has to argue that these children need more one to one therapy, yet the caseload demands force clinicians into working with larger groups of children, often with less progress on the part of each child. The third issue in the schools has come about due to shortages of qualified personnel to serve children in the schools. Consequently, many school systems resort to hiring of unqualified personnel to provide speech-language-hearing services for their students. These personnel are often speech-language pathology students who have a bachelor's degree, but not the master's degree, which is considered by ASHA to be the entry-level degree for the profession. Other personnel functioning as a speech-language pathologist include teachers who are assigned "out of field" for a 1- to 2-year period.

## Model for Clinical Ethical Decision-Making

More and more, in all professional settings in which speech-language pathologists work, ethics affect the clinical decision-making process. Sharp (1998) differentiates between clinical decisions and ethical decisions by writing that clinical decision questions are based on,

"Can we . . . ?" whereas ethical decisions are based on "Should we . . . ?" Four key principles of bioethics need to be considered when making a clinical ethical decision:

1. Autonomy: The right to self-determination, maximizing the patient's independence in clinical decision-making
2. Beneficence: To benefit the patient
3. Nonmaleficence: To "do no harm" to a patient
4. Justice: Fair and equal treatment of patients

Jonsen, Siegler, and Winslade (1992) proposed a model for clinical and ethical decision-making (Table 6–1).

Further explanations by Sharp (1998) of the model include the following:

Medical/Clinical Indications include the clinical and medical facts related to the case, including how certain the clinician(s)

**Table 6–1.** Model for Clinical and Ethical Decision Making

| *Medical/Clinical Indications* | *Patient Preferences* |
|---|---|
| Medical history | Personal history/goals |
| Accurate diagnosis | Religious and personal values |
| Accurate prognosis | Expressed preferences |
| Treatment options | Advance directives |
| | Self assessment of quality of life |
| | Ability to make and communicate decisions |
| *Quality of Life* | *Contextual Features* |
| External assessment of benefits and burdens | Economic (insurance, availability, cost) |
| Subjective judgment | Family preferences |
| Who should decide when the patient cannot? | Legal issues |
| | Burdens on caregivers |
| | Team dynamics |

are of the diagnosis, the patient's prognosis, and what treatment options may be available.

Patient Preferences "incorporate the patient's values, religious beliefs, priorities, and goals for treatment. The patient must be informed to participate in shared decision-making.

In analyzing this model, Sharp (1998) writes that "Most clinical and ethical decisions can be made by balancing the medical indications with the preferences of the patient. These two features have the most weight in ethical decision making and thus are depicted above external assessments of quality of life and other contextual features."

When making a decision, the professionals and patient need first to look at the medical/clinical implications and the patient preferences. If the patient is unable to make a decision based on these two factors, the patient and/or his family should, along with the professionals, look at the quality of life issues and the contextual features.

### *When a Patient Disagrees with the Recommendations*

There are a number of reasons a patient may disagree with the recommendations made by the professionals involved in his or her case. One is that the professional staff may have different goals for the patient (Sharp, 1998). Sometimes this can be frustrating for the professional and the patient. It can be complicated by the fact that, if the discussions are being held soon after the diagnosis, the patient may not be ready to fully recognize the implications of the diagnosis; that is to say, he or she may be in denial or angry about the diagnosis and not fully ready to accept it. In cases such as this, it may behoove the professional staff to hold off the discussions until the patient reaches a point of recognition and acceptance of the implications of his or her illness or injury.

A second factor proposed by Sharp (1998) is the patient's personal experiences with the treatment. He or she may know someone who went through the same or a similar experience who did not do well with a particular treatment plan. Also, in the case of long-standing illnesses or injuries, the patient may have been exposed to a treatment plan earlier in his care that was not successful, was painful, or caused too many side effects to want to renew the treatment.

The patient's assessment of his or her own quality of life is a third reason for disagreement presented by Sharp (1998). The patient

may have expectations of what he or she needs to be able to participate in and accomplish the desired goals that are inconsistent with
the plans he or she has. Again, the level of patient awareness and the
stage of the grief process can have an impact on this factor.

Some patients and/or their families may not have enough information to make decisions that are congruent with those of the medical professionals. This can result from the professionals not wanting
to give out more information than the patient can comprehend and
handle, as well as from the patient's not asking the right questions. The
patient also may lack the capacity to understand what is being said to
him or her and to make a decision regarding his care and prognosis.

## Clinician-Doctor Relationship

There may be occasions when the speech-language pathologist dis-
agrees with a physician's conclusions. Reasons for this conflict may lie
in lack of information, poor communication, and different goals for the
patient (Sharp, 1998). Responses to the conflict may be based on the
clinical setting's hierarchy and power rankings. For example, a patient
with dementia who is residing in a long-term care facility may not, in
the clinicians' belief and experience, benefit from therapy, that is,
have reasonable expectations for improvement. If the clinician treats
such a patient, she or he is violating the ASHA Code of Ethics, which
clearly states that treatment should be provided only when reasonable
improvement can be expected. The long-term care facility's administrator may not be a speech-language pathologist and feel no obligation
to comply with the ASHA Code of Ethics. Thus, based on power, the
clinician may face losing his or her job if he or she does not comply
with the administrator's directives, but face sanction from ASHA if he
or she violates the ASHA Code of Ethics.

In such instances, it may be helpful to have a team with decision-
making capabilities and power to help resolve any differences by
bringing a different perspective to the table. As speech-language pathologists, we have an obligation to the team, the medical staff, and the
patient. However, in most medical settings, the ultimate responsibility
for the care of the patient lies in the hands of the physician. One hopes
having a review team can help to resolve any differences of judgment
that exist among the variety of professionals who are treating the patient.

## Clinician-Patient Relationship

At times, there may be a difference of opinion between the clinician and the patient. Adult patients, and families of children, who have decision-making capacity can refuse treatments. If the patient discharges the clinician, the clinician should document the interaction and decision, and offer contact information where the client can reach you if he or she changes his or her mind. If the clinician wishes to terminate the relationship, he or she is obligated to find a replacement. Patients cannot be abandoned.

## What Happens if the Code of Ethics Is Violated?

It should be pointed out that ASHA's jurisdiction only extends to clinicians who are certified by ASHA. Speech-language pathologists are usually required to obtain a state license as well. Hence, these individuals are responsible for meeting the individual states' requirements for practicing, and any violation of state regulations would be referred to the state licensing agency, not to ASHA. Should a certified speech-language pathologist or audiologist violate the ASHA Code of Ethics, the case would be referred to the ASHA Board of Ethics who "will hear the facts in the case and make a determination as to whether the action is a violation of the Code. The Board can impose sanctions on its members, such as suspension or revocation of the Certificate of Clinical Competence" (Golper & Brown, 2004, p. 63). Sanctions passed down by the ASHA Board of Ethics are published in the *ASHA Leader*, a biweekly newspaper from ASHA.

## Reporting Abuse

One of the most painful and difficult decisions many of us face is when and how to report any abuse of patients that we may observe in the course of our interactions. Following are some guidelines for recognizing and reporting abuse of the elderly and children.

## *Abuse of the Elderly*

Abuse of citizens who are 65 years of age or older has been defined by the American Medical Association as:

> An act or omission which results in harm or threatened harm to the health or welfare of an elderly person. Abuse includes intentional infliction of physical or mental injury; sexual abuse; or withholding of necessary food, clothing, and medical needs of an elderly person by one having the care, custody, or responsibility of an elderly person.

Elder abuse can be any one or combinations of the following:

1. Physical abuse which includes sexual abuse, restraints, beating, or pushing that results in bodily harm or mental distress;
2. Neglect which is defined as depriving the elder of essential care, leading to injury and/or life-threatening conditions;
3. Psychological abuse resulting in mental or emotional distress, including threats, infantilization, harassment, or insults;
4. Financial or material abuse including withholding an elder's Social Security funds, as well as theft of the elder's money or possessions; and
5. Violation of constitutional rights such as a right to privacy, the rights of personal property, personal freedom, voting, and free speech (Dikengil, 1998).

Adult Protective Services (APS), as cited by Dikengil (1998), lists signs that an adult may be a victim of abuse:

1. Patient displays a noticeable change in behavior
2. Patient appears to be fearful of the caregiver
3. Patient is reluctant to answer when questioned
4. Caregiver is indifferent or angry toward the patient
5. Caregiver refuses to give necessary assistance to the clinician or patient
6. Caregiver tries to prevent the patient from speaking privately with the clinician (Dikengil, 1998, p. 259)

Other indications that an adult is being abused include factors such as displaying bruises or other injuries, living in a home that has inadequate supplies of food and other essentials, or living in a home that is unsafe, dirty, and/or uncared for.

Most victims of elder abuse are abused by a relative. Relatives who have a history of alcohol or drug abuse, psychological problems, and/or who have difficulty dealing with stress and controlling their anger are more likely to abuse any elderly individuals in their care. Caring for an individual with chronic deficits can be time consuming and stress producing. In addition to monitoring the elderly client for signs of abuse, the clinician should also observe the caregiver for any of these symptoms. If the caregiver is expressing signs of stress, anger, or depression, he or she should be referred for psychological or psychiatric evaluation and treatment. Pollick (1987) states that abuse of the elderly can be prevented if we, as health care practitioners, educate their families about problems elderly people face, and provide the caregivers options they can pursue for assistance in caring for their elderly family member(s).

### *Abuse of Children*

The second highest cause of death in children is abuse. (Purdum & Trudel, as cited in Dikengil, 1998). Dikengil describes behaviors often seen in children who have been abused and/or neglected:

1. wariness of adult contact
2. fear of parents or fear of going/being home
3. extreme aggression or withdrawal
4. delinquency or stealing
5. falling asleep; nightmares
6. alcohol or drug abuse
7. unwilling to change for gym class
8. poor peer relationships
9. inappropriate knowledge of sexual behavior
10. fecal smearing
11. behavior extremes
12. attempted suicide (p. 261).

Most states require educators and health care personnel to report suspected child abuse. Educators are of particular interest because they are the largest group of individuals who work with children. Referrals may be made anonymously, if so chosen. Suspicion of child abuse or neglect is adequate ground for making a referral. Educators are not responsible for proving that a child is a victim of neglect or abuse, but they can report it when it is suspected.

According to the Health and Rehabilitative Services Protection Team, the following are signs of child abuse and/or neglect:

A. Physical Abuse:
   1. Bruises and welts in various stages of healing
   2. Burns that show the shape of an item used to inflict them (cigarette tip, iron, grill, etc.); rope burns
   3. Human bite marks
   4. Reports of injury by caretaker (from child or friend)
   5. Parent or child attempts to conceal injury or offers illogical, unconvincing, contradictory or no explanation of the child's injury
   6. Fractures in various stages of healing

B. Neglect/Emotional Maltreatment:
   1. Child consistently dirty, unwashed, hungry, or inappropriately dressed
   2. Child without supervision for long periods of time
   3. Child has unattended physical problems
   4. Child constantly tired or listless
   5. Child rarely attends school
   6. Child exhibits behavioral problems (overly compliant, lags in emotional development, attempts suicide)

C. Sexual Abuse
   1. Child has stained, torn, or bloody underclothing
   2. Child has venereal disease
   3. Child is pregnant
   4. Child experiences pain or itching in genital area
   5. Child has bruises, laceration or semen around genital areas or mouth
   6. Child is unwilling to participate in physical activities.

Adults who abuse children have many of the same characteristics as those who abuse adults, in addition to marital difficulties and being young and/or single with children.

There is a national hot line that can be called to report suspected abuse or neglect of a child. The hotline's number is 1-800-4-A-CHILD

(1-800-422-4453). After dialing, push 1 to talk with a counselor. This number can be called by residents of the United States, Canada, Puerto Rico, or the U.S. Virgin Islands. It can be called 24 hours a day, 7 days a week. The caller can remain anonymous, and there is no charge for the call. Hotline counselors can access a database containing social service, emergency, and support resources.

## Summary

In an effort to find out some of the real-world ethical issues faced by speech-language pathologists, the author conducted a survey of practicum supervisors in a variety of settings. Clearly, we face a wide variety of possible dilemmas in our various places of work. These are summarized in Table 6–2. The reader is encouraged to review this list and ethics education materials available from ASHA to know learn how to avoid, face, and report ethical situations/occurrences.

**Table 6–2.** Ethical Dilemmas Faced in Different Work Settings (Based on Author's Survey of Practicing Clinicians)

| |
|---|
| **Hospital-Affiliated Outpatient Clinic** |
| Recommending NPO |
| Seeing unethical practices around you and knowing what to do about it |
| Dealing with supervisors who are unethical about billing |
| Confidentiality because in an outpatient setting family and friends who transport patients to therapy feel as though they can join the patient in therapy. |
| **Acute-Care Hospital** |
| A boss who expected me to keep the patients beyond the point they needed to be seen |
| None specifically due to taking a strong stance against negative changes although the hospital attempted to increase rates to a point I felt was overbilling. I documented my disagreement through e-mail communications |
| Knowing how to handle unethical situations around me |

**Table 6–2.** *continued*

### University Clinic

Balancing a client's need for continued treatment versus the students' needs for clock hours

Working with a clinician who speaks English as a second language who is not proficient in English but is supposed to learn to provide therapy

Blame being placed on workers when jobs are misunderstood by management

Being required to do an evaluation of a type of client that I was not trained for

Concerned about scope of practice being followed by co-workers at all times

Seeing peers being unethical and not being comfortable reporting them

Knowing when and to whom to report parents who do not fulfill their responsibilities with regard to their child/children's care

Staying current in every area you work in

### Elementary School

Photocopying of copyrighted materials due to low budgets

Being asked to make a "school" decision versus what I know is the right thing to do

Carrying out effective evidence-based therapy

### Private Practice

Whether or not to continue providing therapy to patients who have shown no progress over several evaluation periods

### Community Clinic

A home health patient really needs treatment but does not really meet home care criteria

As we are a child-focused program, and a lot of the parents are friends, I am constantly facing the issue of parents inquiring about another child in the program. I am always having to tell parents that even though they are close with another one of my patients, I cannot tell them how another child is doing in therapy

# References

American Speech Language Hearing Association. (2003). *Code of ethics.* Rockville, MD: Author.

Dikengil, A. T. (1998). *Handbook of home health care for the speech-language pathologist.* San Diego, CA: Singular.

Golper, L. A. C., & Brown, J. E. (2004). *Business matters: A guide for speech-language pathologists.* Rockville, MD: American Speech-Language-Hearing Association.

Harris, C. E., Jr. (1986). *Applying moral theories.* Belmont, CA: Wadsworth.

Jonsen, A. R., Siegler, M., & Winslade, W. J. (1992). *Clinical ethics: A practical approach to ethical decisions in clinical medicine* (3rd ed.). New York: McGraw-Hill.

Lubinski, R., & Frattali, C. (1994). *Professional issues in speech-language pathology and audiology: A textbook.* San Diego, CA: Singular.

Pollick, M. F. (1987). Abuse of the elderly: A review. *Holistic Nursing Practice,* pp. 43–53.

Resnick, D. M. (1993). *Professional ethics for audiologists and speech-language pathologists.* San Diego, CA: Singular.

Seymour, C. M. (1994). Ethical considerations. In R. Lubinski & C. Frattali, *Professional issues in speech-language pathology and audiology: A textbook.* San Diego, CA: Singular.

Sharp, H. M. (1998, January). *Ethics, healthcare, and speech-language pathology.* Presentation at Florida Speech-Language-Hearing Association Winter Convention. Gainesville, FL.

Solomon, R. C. (1984). *Ethics: A brief introduction.* New York: McGraw-Hill.

# APPENDIX 6A
## ASHA Code of Ethics (2003)

## *Preamble*

The preservation of the highest standards of integrity and ethical principles is vital to the responsible discharge of obligations by speech-language pathologists, audiologists, and speech, language, hearing scientists. This Code of Ethics sets forth the fundamental principles and rules considered essential to this purpose.

Every individual who is (a) a member of the American Speech-Language-Hearing Association, whether certified or not, (b) a nonmember holding the Certificate of Clinical Competence from the Association, (c) an applicant for membership or certification, or (d) a Clinical Fellow seeking to fulfill standards of certification shall abide by this Code of Ethics.

Any violation of the spirit and purpose of this Code shall be considered unethical. Failure to specify any particular responsibility or practice in this Code of Ethics shall not be construed as denial of the existence of such responsibilities or practices.

The fundamentals of ethical conduct are described by the Principles of Ethics and by Rules of Ethics as they relate to the conduct of research and scholarly activities and responsibility to persons served, the public, and speech-language pathologists, audiologists, and speech, language, and hearing scientists.

Principles of Ethics, aspirational and inspirational in nature, form the underlying moral basis for the Code of Ethics. Individuals shall observe these principles as affirmative obligations under all conditions or professional activity.

Rules of Ethics are specific statements of minimally acceptable professional conduct or of prohibitions and are applicable to all individuals.

## *Principle of Ethics I*

Individuals shall honor their responsibility to hold paramount the welfare of persons they serve professionally or participants in research and scholarly activities and shall treat animals involved in research in a humane manner.

## Rules of Ethics

**A.** Individuals shall provide all services competently.

**B.** Individuals shall use every resource including referral when appropriate, to ensure the high-quality service is provided.

**C.** Individuals shall not discriminate in the delivery of professional services or the conduct of research and scholarly activities on the basis of race, ethnicity, gender, age, religion, national origin, sexual orientation, or disability.

**D.** Individuals shall not misrepresent the credentials of assistants, technicians, or support personnel and shall inform those they serve professionally of the name and professional credentials of the persons providing services.

**E.** Individuals who hold the Certificates of Clinical Competence shall not delegate tasks that require the unique skills, knowledge, and judgment that are within the scope of their profession to assistants, technicians, support personnel, students, or any nonprofessionals over whom they have supervisory responsibility. An individual may delegate students, or any nonprofessionals over whom they have supervisory responsibility. An individual may delegate support services to assistants, technicians, support personnel, students, or any other persons only if those services are adequately supervised by an individual who holds the appropriate Certificate of Clinical Competence.

**F.** Individuals shall fully inform the persons they serve of the nature and possible effects of services rendered and products dispensed, and they shall inform participants in research about the possible effects of their participation in research conducted.

**G.** Individuals shall evaluate the effectiveness of services rendered and or products dispensed and shall provide services or dispense products only when benefit can reasonably be expected.

**H.** Individuals shall not guarantee the results of any treatment or procedure, directly or by implication; however, they may make a reasonable state of prognosis

**I.** Individuals shall not provide clinical services solely by correspondence.

**J.** Individuals may practice by telecommunication (for example, telehealth/e-health) where not prohibited by law.

**K.** Individuals shall adequately maintain and appropriately secure records of professional services rendered, research and scholarly activities conducted, and products dispensed and shall allow access to these records only when authorized or when required by law.

**L.** Individuals shall not reveal, without authorization, any professional or personal information about identified persons served professionally, identified participants involved in research and scholarly activities unless required by law to do so, or unless doing so is necessary to protect the welfare of the person or of the community or otherwise required by law

**M.** Individuals shall not charge for services not rendered, nor shall they misrepresent services rendered, products dispensed, or research and scholarly activities conducted.

**N.** Individuals shall use persons in research or as subjects of teaching demonstrations only with their informed consent.

**O.** Individuals whose professional services are adversely affected by substance abuse or other health-related conditions shall seek professional assistance, and, where appropriate, withdraw from the affected areas of practice.

## *Principle of Ethics II*

Individuals shall honor their responsibility to achieve and maintain the highest level of professional competence.

### Rules of Ethics

**A.** Individuals shall engage in the provision of clinical services only when they hold the appropriate Certificate of Clinical Competence or when they are in the certification process and are supervised by an individual who holds the appropriate Certificate of Clinical Competence.

**B.** Individuals shall engage in only those aspects of the professions that are within the scope of their competence, considering their level of education, training, and experience.

**C.** Individuals shall continue their professional development throughout their careers.

**D.** Individuals shall delegate the provision of clinical services only to: (1) persons who hold the appropriate Certificate of Clinical Competence; (2) persons in the education or certification process who are appropriately supervised by an individual who holds the appropriate Certificate of Clinical Competence; or (3) assistants, technicians, or support personnel who are adequately supervised by an individual who holds the appropriate Certificate of Clinical Competence.

**E.** Individuals shall not require or permit their professional staff to provide services or conduct research activities that exceed the staff member's competence, level of education, training, and experience.

**F.** Individuals shall ensure that all equipment used in the provision of services or to conduct research and scholarly activities is in proper working order and is properly calibrated.

## *Principle of Ethics III*

Individuals shall honor their responsibility to the public by promoting public understanding of the professions, by supporting the development of services designed to fulfill the unmet needs of the public, and by providing accurate information in all communications involving any aspect of the professions, including dissemination of research findings and scholarly activities.

## Rules of Ethics

**A.** Individuals shall not misrepresent their credentials, competence, education, training, experience, or scholarly or research contributions.

**B.** Individuals shall not participate in professional activities that constitute a conflict of interest.

**C.** Individuals shall refer those served professionally solely on the basis of the interest of those being referred and not on any personal financial interest.

**D.** Individuals shall not misrepresent diagnostic information, research, services rendered, or products dispensed; neither shall they engage in any scheme to defraud in connection with obtaining payment or reimbursement for such services or products.

**E.** Individuals' statements to the public shall provide accurate information about the nature and management of communication disorders about the professions, about professional services, and about research and scholarly activities.

**F.** Individuals' statements to the public—advertising, announcing, and marketing their professional services, reporting research results, and promoting products—shall adhere to prevailing professional standards ad shall not contain misrepresentations.

## *Principles of Ethics IV*

Individuals shall honor their responsibilities to the professions and their relationships with colleagues, students, and members of allied professions. Individuals shall uphold the dignity and autonomy of the professions, maintain harmonious interprofessional and intraprofessional relationships, and accept the professions' self-imposed standards.

### Rules of Ethics

**A.** Individuals shall prohibit anyone under their supervision from engaging in any practice that violates the Code of Ethics.

**B.** Individuals shall not engage in dishonesty, fraud, deceit, misrepresentation, sexual harassment, or any other form of conduct that adversely reflects on the professions or on the individual's fitness to serve persons professionally.

**C.** Individuals shall not engage in sexual activities with clients or students over whom they exercise professional authority

**D.** Individuals shall assign credit only to those who have contributed to a publication, presentation, or product. Credit shall be assigned in proportion to the contribution and only with the contributor's consent.

**E.** Individuals shall reference the source when using other people's ideas, research, presentations, or products in written, oral, or any other media presentation or summary.

**F.** Individuals' statements to colleagues about professional services, research results, and products shall adhere to prevailing professional standards and shall contain no misrepresentations.

**G.** Individuals shall not provide professional services without exercising independent professional judgment, regardless of referral source or prescription.

**H.** Individuals shall not discriminate in their relationships with colleagues, students, and members of allied professionals on the basis of race or ethnicity, gender, age, religion, national origin, sexual orientation, or disability.

**I.** Individuals who have reason to believe that the Code of Ethics has been violated shall inform the Board of Ethics.

**J.** Individuals shall comply fully with the policies of the Board of Ethics in its consideration and adjudication of complaints of violations of the Code of Ethics.

---

# *Chapter 7*

# Professional Standards

Standards exist as quality assurance mechanisms to protect the consumer and to ensure quality services and quality products. ASHA sets three types of standards for the following:

1. The provision of services by individuals to persons with communication disorders.
2. The provision of services by programs to persons with communication disorders.
3. The graduate education of persons providing the services.

Standards are needed to help consumers determine the equality of services and products. It is better to develop standards internally as much as possible. Otherwise, external groups may develop standards without having adequate understanding of all the issues involved in developing standards that are in the best interest of the consumer, and standards that place reasonable requirements on the service provider.

Standards include policies and procedures. A policy is defined as "broad, current, comprehensive, inviolate (statements) written to specify responsibility for action" (Bureau of Business Practices, 1988). Procedures are sequences of steps needed to complete a specific activity. Procedures may change frequently; policies are more long-term in nature. A policy and procedure manual is a "consistent guide to be followed under a given set of circumstances" (Rao & Goldsmith, 1994, in Lubinsky & Frattali, p. 233). The manual serves as a framework for management and staff decision making and it organizes and centralizes the policies and procedures governing an organization. It is suggested that the content of a policy and procedure manual in a speech-language pathology practice follow the eight mandatory areas for review for accreditation by what was formerly known as the Professional Services Board:

1. Missions, goals, and objectives;
2. Nature and quality of services;
3. Quality improvement and program evaluation (effectiveness and efficiency of services provided);
4. Administration (licensure, leave, federal, state, and local regulations);
5. Financial resources and management;
6. Human resources (continuing education);
7. Physical facilities and program environment; and
8. Equipment and materials.

In the spring of 2001, the ASHA Legislative Council dissolved the Council for Professional Services Accreditation (CPSA) and the accreditation of programs providing audiology and/or speech-language pathology services. The standards the CPSA developed were approved in 2000 by the ASHA Standards Council and put into effect in January 2002. These standards, called "quality indicators," were to help professional services programs to identify and describe indicators of quality, to assist programs in self-evaluation activities, and to provide a guide for the development of policies and procedures to facilitate provision of quality professional services. At the same Legislative Council meeting, a resolution was passed to "develop and disseminate quality indicators by January, 2005." The document was to be disseminated to programs providing audiology and speech-language pathology services as a resource to assist service programs. It should be noted that, although the 2002 standards are mandatory, the quality indicators document are guidelines, not requirements. The quality indicators apply to all settings and include purpose and scope of services, service delivery, program operation, program evaluation and performance improvement. (ASHA, 2005).

For members of the American Speech-Language-Hearing Association, standards are developed by two councils: the Council on Academic Accreditation in Audiology and Speech-Language Pathology (accredits academic graduate programs dedicated to the preparation of speech-language pathologists and audiologists), and the Council for Clinical Certification in Audiology and Speech-Language Pathology.

Accreditation of graduate programs by the Council on Academic Accreditation (CAA) is based on a review of six areas: (1) structure and governance, (2) faculty, (3) curriculum, (4) students, (5) assessment, and (6) program resources. Site visit teams consisting of three to four members visit each graduate program every seven years to review the status of the program. The site visit team writes a report in which they state their ability to determine compliance with all the standards set forth by CAA. This report is then filed with the CAA who determines whether or not to accredit the graduate program. Universities have a chance to respond to any concerns stated by the site visit team; this response is also considered by the CAA in making its determination with regard to accreditation of that graduate program.

## CARF: Commission on Accreditation of Rehabilitation Facilities

CARF began in 1966 as a not-for-profit, private commission for the accreditation of rehabilitation facilities. It is a commission that functions as an international (Canada, Europe, South America, United States) rehabilitation accreditation agency for rehabilitation organizations including Speech-Language Pathology, Physical Therapy, Occupational Therapy, Vocational Rehabilitation, Recreation Therapy, Music Therapy, and Psychological Counseling.

Accountability and quality are the objectives CARF strives to meet. However, their approach allows the care agency seeking CARF accreditation to incorporate CARF's standards into practices and policies that reflect the vision, mission, and identity as a provider of rehabilitation services.

CARF accreditation is a public acknowledgement that the rehabilitation facility bearing CARF accreditation "strives to improve efficiency, fiscal health, and service delivery—creating a foundation for continuous quality improvement and consumer satisfaction" (http://www.carf.org). Given these commitments that seem to be at the core of CARF accredited agencies, governmental regulators, insurers, and third-party payers are more likely to view CARF-accredited services as a worthy risk. Ultimately, the "greatest value is assuring the persons you serve, and their families, that your services are focused on their unique needs"(http://www.carf.org).

**The Aging Services customer service unit** focuses on service areas serving older adults across the continuum. In 2003, the Continuing

Care Accreditation Commission (CCAC) combined with CARF; together they are the only accrediting commission for networks of aging services, including Continuing Care Retirement Communities (CCRCs). Providers may become accredited in one or more program areas. The specific areas are adult day care facilities, assisted living centers, continuing care retirement communities which use the CARF-CCAC accreditation program, nursing homes (person-centered long-term care communities), and comprehensive integrated inpatient rehabilitation programs. In any of the settings listed in the previous paragraph, providers also may pursue a specialization in stroke programs and dementia care.

**Behavioral Health** programs include services to persons or families with needs related to mental illness, alcohol or other drug usage, and other addictions, such as gambling. The services may address relationship or adjustment concerns, domestic violence, and other family issues. The services may be designed to prevent potential problems and treat existing ones. Behavioral health programs are provided in a variety of settings ranging from clinics and inpatient locations to the home, school, community, or criminal justice settings.

**DMEPOS** refers to Durable Medical Equipment, Prosthetics, Orthotics, and Supplies. This agreement was made in 2006 and fully implemented in February 2007. CARF works with the Centers for Medicare and Medicaid Services (CMS) in its efforts to ensure that Medicare beneficiaries have access to high quality DMEPOS and related services.

**Child and Youth Services** (CYS) programs provide child welfare, protection, and well-being services to children, youths, and their families. Opportunities are maximized for the children/youths served to obtain and participate in the services. Services are provided with recognition that the family (birth, extended, or placement) is the constant in the child's life.

Parent/professional collaboration is facilitated at all levels of care with the understanding and incorporation of the strengths and needs of infants, children, and youths and their families into the service systems. CYS programs are provided in a variety of settings, ranging from clinics and residential facilities to home, school, community, or juvenile justice settings.

**Employment and Community Services** help people gain skills or supports needed to work and live where they choose. Employment Services help individuals pursue their employment plans, get training if needed, and find employment in a job of their choice. Community

Services help people with a wide variety of needs to receive the services they want and choose so that they can participate more independently in their communities. These services might be options of various living arrangements, participation in day programs and community activities, and support for caregivers, foster families, or host families.

**Assistive Technology Services** help persons in making informed decisions and choices in selection and use of assistive technology devices to increase employment options, independence, and inclusion in the community.

**Vision Rehabilitation Services** provide a comprehensive rehabilitation program, including skills acquisition, psychosocial adjustment, and community reentry.

**Medical Rehabilitation** programs include treatments for people who have had a stroke, brain or spinal cord injury, or pain that cannot be controlled by medication alone. Medical rehabilitation also includes return-to-work programs or occupational rehabilitation, which helps people regain skills they need so that they can return to work after an injury or illness. Medical rehabilitation services might be provided in a hospital, an outpatient clinic, an individual's home, the work site, or other settings in the community. Medical Rehabilitation programs may serve specific age groups (such as children and adolescents or adults) or all ages.

## *Condensed Steps to Accreditation (from the CARF standards manuals)*

The steps to accreditation involve a year or more of preparation before the site survey and ongoing quality improvement following the survey. Following is a condensed version of the CARF standards. One can go on-line to http://www.carf.org or the CARF standards manuals to find more information about each item.

1. **Consult with a designated CARF resource specialist** to provide guidance and technical assistance regarding the accreditation process.

2. **Conduct a self-evaluation.** The organization must implement and use the standards for at least six months before the survey.

3. **Submit the Intent to Survey and nonrefundable intent fee.** The intent survey includes detailed information about leadership,

programs, and services that the organization is seeking to accredit and the service delivery location(s).

4. **CARF invoices for the survey fee.** The CARF fee is based on the number of surveyors and days needed to complete the survey. The CARF-CCAC fee is fixed, with additional fees if more programs are added to the survey.

5. **CARF selects the survey team.** Surveyors are selected by matching their program or administrative expertise and relevant field experience with the organization's unique requirements.

6. **The survey team conducts the survey** and determines the organization's conformance to all applicable standards on site by observing services, interviewing persons served and other stakeholders, and reviewing documentation. Surveyors also provide consultation to organization personnel.

7. **CARF renders an accreditation outcome.** CARF reviews the survey findings and renders one of the following accreditation decisions:

CARF

- Three-year accreditation
- One-year accreditation
- Provisional accreditation
- Nonaccreditation

CARF-CCAC

- Five-year term of accreditation
- Nonaccreditation (www.carf.org).

Approximately 6 to 8 weeks after the survey, CARF notifies the organization of the accreditation outcome and sends it a written survey report and Quality Improvement Plan (QIP).

8. **Submit a Quality Improvement Plan (QIP).** Within 90 days after notification of the accreditation outcome, the organization fulfills an accreditation condition by submitting to CARF a QIP outlining the actions that have been or will be taken in response to the recommendations made in the survey report.

    CARF-CCAC-accredited organizations must also submit a QIP with the Annual Conformance to Quality Report (ACQR).

9. **Submit an Annual Conformance to Quality Report.** An organization that earns accreditation submits to CARF a signed ACQR

on the accreditation anniversary date in each of the years following the award.

10. **CARF maintains contact with the organization** during the accreditation tenure. Organizations are also encouraged to contact CARF as needed to help maintain conformance to CARF standards. (Copyright CARF © 2007. All rights reserved. Reprinted with permission)

### *Contact Information*

CARF International
4891 E. Grant Road
Tucson, AZ 85712 USA
(520) 325-1044 or toll-free (888) 281-6531 voice/TTY
(520) 318-1129 Fax

CARF Canada
10665 Jasper Avenue, Suite 1400A
Edmonton, AB T5J 3S9 Canada
(780) 429-2538 or toll-free (877) 434-5444 voice
(780) 426-7274 Fax
or Ottawa, Ontario, call (613) 726-7922

CARF-CCAC
1730 Rhode Island Avenue NW, Suite 209
Washington, DC 20036 USA
(202) 587-5001 or toll-free (866) 888-1122 voice
(202) 587-5009 Fax

## The Joint Commission (Formerly Known as the Joint Commission on Accreditation of Healthcare Organizations [JCAHO])

### *Position Statement: Helping Health Care Organizations Help Patients*

The Joint Commission is a nonprofit, independent organization that accredits health care agencies throughout the United States. Its mission is "to continuously improve the safety and quality of care provided to the pubic through the provision of health care accreditation and related services that support performance improvement in health care organizations" (JCAHO Web site, 2005).

The Joint Commission is governed by "a 29-member Board of Commissioners that includes physicians, administrators, nurses, employers, a labor representative, health plan leaders, quality experts, ethicists, a consumer advocate and educators. The Joint Commission's corporate members are the American College of Physicians, the American College of Surgeons, the American Dental Association, the American Hospital Association, and the American Medical Association. The Joint Commission employs approximately 1,000 people in its surveyor force at its central office in Oakbrook Terrace, Illinois, and at a satellite office in Washington, D.C. The Washington office is The Joint Commission's primary interface with government agencies and with Congress, seeking and maintaining partnerships with the government that will improve the quality of health care for all Americans, and working with Congress on legislation involving the quality and safety of health care" (JCAHO Web site, retrieved 10/25/07)

The Joint Commission accredits approximately 15,000 health care organizations in the United States, including the following types:

Ambulatory care providers

Behavioral health organizations (addiction services)

Clinical laboratories

Health care networks

Home care organizations (including hospice services)

Hospitals

    acute-care hospitals

    children's hospitals

    critical access hospitals

    psychiatric hospitals

    rehabilitation hospitals/centers

Long-term care facilities

Medical equipment services

Skilled nursing facilities

With the exception of clinical laboratories that must be surveyed by a team from the Joint Commission every two years, facilities must have a site visit and apply for reaccreditation every three years.

In addition to accreditation, the Joint Commission awards Disease-Specific Care Certification to health plans, disease management service companies, hospitals, and other care delivery settings that provide disease management and chronic care services. The Joint Commission also has a Health Care Staffing Services Certification Program and is developing a certification program for transplant centers and health care services. The Joint Commission develops its standards in consultation with health care experts, providers, measurement experts, purchasers, and consumers. Disease-Specific-Care Certification Programs include the following:

Chronic kidney disease

Chronic obstructive pulmonary disease (COPD)

Inpatient diabetes

Lung volume reduction surgery

Primary stroke centers

Transplant center

Ventricular assist device

Certification programs also include health care staffing services (JCAHO Web site, retrieved 10/25/07)

Historically, accreditation from JCAHO focused on policies and procedures addressing patient safety, service issues, and clinical quality. In other words, what is the actual experience a patient has when in one of the above settings? As part of the evaluation of patient care, Joint Commission assesses the communication between members of patient care teams, the rights and ethics of the patient in the facility, the monitoring of quality of services, the state of the facility (including cleanliness), and information management. With regard to quality of services, emphasis is placed on how well the facility achieves the goals set forth by the Institute of Medicine:

Safety

Effective (evidence-based practice)

Patient-centered care

Timeliness of care being provided

Efficiency

Equal care (with regard to ethnic origin, geographic location, gender, or socioeconomics status) (Lubinski, Golper, & Frattali, 2007).

It is advantageous for health care organizations to seek accreditation and certification by the Joint Commission. Specifically, the organizations can expect to reap the following benefits:

- Strengthens community confidence in the quality and safety of care, treatment, and services
- Provides a competitive edge in the marketplace
- Improves risk management and risk reduction
- Provides education on good practices to improve business operations
- Provides professional advice and counsel, enhancing staff education
- Enhances staff recruitment and development
- Recognized by select insurers and other third parties
- May fulfill regulatory requirements in select states (JCAHO Web site, retrieved 10/25/07)

The Joint Commission standards address the organization's level of performance in key functional areas, such as patient rights, patient treatment, and infection control. A health care organization is not accredited for its "ability to provide safe, high quality care, but on its actual performance as well with the safety and quality of patient care being of most concern" (JCAHO Web site, retrieved 10/25/07). When the agency is granted accreditation by the Joint Commission, it receives the "Gold Seal of Approval."

The "2008 National Patient Safety Goals/Hospital Program" can be found in Appendix 7A.

### Contact Information

The Joint Commission
One Renaissance Boulevard

Oakbrook Terrace, IL 60181
(708)916-5400
http://www.jointcommission.org

## National Committee for Quality Assurance

The National Committee for Quality Assurance (NCQA) serves as the accrediting agency for managed care organizations and preferred provider organizations. It also develops outcome measures.

## Summary

As a professional speech-language pathologist, you are expected to exercise more than reasonable care, and this is defined by ASHA's standard of accepted professional practice. Standards of care defined by statutory laws are those created by federal, state, or local legislative bodies. Licensure laws and laws defining the scope of practice fall under the jurisdiction of statutory laws.

Standards of care defined by common law include those that are created as the result of principles that are established through the resolution of prior legal actions. Finally, standards of care defined by the ASHA Code of Ethics define such things as proper evaluation, proper treatment, and appropriate referrals.

ASHA publishes standards of care that outline the reasonable measures that should be taken in the care of patients of speech-language pathologists and audiologists. According to Scott (2000), there are three formulations for the legal standard of care for health care professionals:

1. Traditional rule: Compare the health care professionals with peers in the same community.
2. Modern majority rule: Compare the health care professional with peers in the same community or in similar communities, state- or nationwide.
3. Trend: Compare the health care professional with any or all peers, state- or nationwide, acting under the same or similar circumstances (p. 8).

Standards of care are defined nationally by various accrediting agencies, as well as locally by the facilities serving the patients. The speech-language pathologist is responsible for knowing, abiding by, and upholding the standards of care that are in effect in any facility in which he or she works.

# References

American Speech-Language-Hearing Association. (2005). *Quality indicators for professional service programs in audiology and speech-language pathology.* Rockville, MD: Author.

Bureau of Businss Practice. (1988). *Personnel policy manual.* Englewood Cliffs, NJ: Prentice-Hall.

Commission on Accreditation of Rehabilitation Facilities (CARF). http://www.carf.org

Joint Commission on Accreditation of Health Care Organizations (JCAHCO). (2007). *Position statement: Helping Health Care Organizations help patients.* Retrieved 10/25/07 from: http://www.jointcommission.org/standards

Lubinski, R., Golper, L. A. C., & Frattali, C. M. (2007). *Professional issues in speech-language pathology and audiology* (3rd ed.). Clifton Park, NY: Thomson Delmar Learning.

Rao, P., & Goldsmith, T. (1994). Developing policies and procedures. In R. Lubinski & C. Frattali (Eds.), *Professional issues in speech-language pathology and audiology* (pp. 233–245). San Diego, CA: Singular.

Scott, R. W. (2000). *Legal aspects of documenting patient care* (2nd ed.). Gaithersburg, MD: Aspen.

# APPENDIX 7A
## 2008 National Patient Safety Goals
## Hospital Program

2008 National Patient Safety Goals Manual Chapter
(Includes Rationales and Implementation Expectations)

Note: Changes to the Goals and Requirements are indicated in **bold.** Gaps in the numbering indicate that the Goal is inapplicable to the program or has been "retired," usually because the requirements were integrated into the standards.

**This year's new requirements (3E and 16A) have a one-year phase-in period that includes defined expectations for planning, development and testing ("milestones") at 3, 6 and 9 months in 2008, with the expectation of full implementation by January 2009. See the Implementation Expectations for milestones.**

| | |
|---|---|
| Goal 1 | Improve the accuracy of patient identification. |
| 1A | Use at least two patient identifiers when providing care, treatment or services. |
| Goal 2 | Improve the effectiveness of communication among caregivers. |
| 2A | For verbal or telephone orders or for telephonic reporting of critical test results, verify the complete order or test result by having the person receiving the information record and "read-back" the complete order or test result. |
| 2B | Standardize a list of abbreviations, acronyms, symbols, and dose designations that are to be used throughout the organization. |
| 2C | Measure and assess and, if appropriate, take action to improve the timeliness of reporting, and the timeliness of receipt by the responsible licensed caregiver, of critical test results and values. |
| 2E | Implement a standardized approach to "hand off" communications, including an opportunity to ask and respond to questions. |

| | |
|---|---|
| Goal 3 | Improve the safety of using medications. |
| 3C | Identify and, at a minimum, annually review a list of look-alike/sound-alike drugs used by the organization, and take action to prevent errors involving the interchange of these drugs. |
| 3D | Label all medications, medication containers (for example, syringes, medicine cups, basins), or other solutions on and off the sterile field. |
| **3E** | **Reduce the likelihood of patient harm associated with the use of anticoagulation therapy.** |
| Goal 7 | Reduce the risk of health care-associated infections. |
| 7A | Comply with current **World Health Organization (WHO) Hand Hygiene Guidelines** or Centers for Disease Control and Prevention (CDC) hand hygiene guidelines. |
| 7B | Manage as sentinel events all identified cases of unanticipated death or major permanent loss of function associated with a health care-associated infection. |
| Goal 8 | Accurately and completely reconcile medications across the continuum of care. |
| 8A | There is a process for comparing the patient's current medications with those ordered for the patient while under the care of the organization. |
| 8B | A complete list of the patient's medications is communicated to the next provider of service when a patient is referred or transferred to another setting, service, practitioner or level of care within or outside the organization. The complete list of medications is also provided to the patient on discharge from the facility. |
| Goal 9 | Reduce the risk of patient harm resulting from falls. |
| 9B | Implement a fall reduction program including an evaluation of the effectiveness of the program. |
| Goal 13 | Encourage patients' active involvement in their own care as a patient safety strategy. |

13A     Define and communicate the means for patients and their
        families to report concerns about safety and encourage
        them to do so.

Goal 15 The organization identifies safety risks inherent in its
        patient population.

15A     The organization identifies patients at risk for suicide.
        [Applicable to psychiatric hospitals and patients being
        treated for emotional or behavioral disorders in general
        hospitals—NOT APPLICABLE TO CRITICAL ACCESS
        HOSPITALS)]

**Goal 16 Improve recognition and response to changes in a
        patient's condition.**

**16A    The organization selects a suitable method that
        enables health care staff members to directly
        request additional assistance from a specially
        trained individual(s) when the patient's condition
        appears to be worsening. [Critical Access Hospital,
        Hospital]**

---

*Source:* Joint Commission on Accreditation of Hospitals. Reprinted with permission.

# SECTION III

## Workplace Skills

# Chapter 8

# Clinical Decision-Making

*"If you want to succeed, you must take responsibility and make choices."*

(Kreuger, 1995, p. 79)

*"The problem with decisions is that they are made in the present, analyzed by past information, to be acted upon in the future!"*

(Kreuger, 1995, p. 86)

## Introduction

Butler and Hope (1995) have summarized several myths about decision-making. The two most prevalent are that (1) everything depends on reaching the right decision, and (2) "people are either decisive or indecisive" (p. 386). The purpose of this chapter is to minimize the myths, minimize the fear of making decisions, and maximize those skills that enable us to make a decision that is appropriate, reasonable, and justifiable given current evidence.

## Steps to Minimize the Fear of Making Decisions

We all know someone who cannot make a decision without much trepidation. This can range from something as simple as, "Do I buy the red shirt or the blue shirt?" to something major such as "Do we take this person off life support, or do we leave him on life support?" For many people, fear of making a decision is a major factor, sometimes to the point of not making the decision at all for fear of making the wrong one. Cynthia Kreuger (1995) lists four steps to be followed to help minimize the fear of making decisions:

1. Make a list of pros and cons of all possible decisions
2. Look to more experienced colleagues for advice
3. Use other coworkers as sounding boards
4. Come up with a strong case for one side

If one takes time to work through these four steps, he or she can make a more reasoned and justifiable decision, and hopefully achieve some sense of satisfaction that the correct decision has been made. However, there are also dangers in decision making, also listed by Kreuger:

1. Procrastination
2. Letting someone else take over
3. Relying on habit

By procrastinating on making a decision, one may find that the decision is made by time. How many times have you heard, "Well, it's too late now," as a comment when a person has put off making a decision? In a professional setting, in particular, procrastinating in the decision-making process may send a message that you are lazy, unconcerned, and/or irresponsible. Procrastination should not be confused with setting aside a project or decision in an effort to look at the dilemma from a fresh perspective (Kreuger, 1995). This action sometimes leads to a more thought-out, justifiable decision than making a rash conclusion in the interest of being a servant to time.

Just as procrastinating can leave a negative impression of incompetence in the professional setting, so can allowing others to make decisions for you. "If you allow others to make decisions for you, you may lose credibility. People will feel they can't count on you and you'll be thought of as wishy-washy and ineffective" (Kreuger, 1995, p. 81).

With regard to relying on habit, there is something to be said for taking into consideration strategies that have worked in the past, and that still may be useful. However, one must remember that there are situations in which it may be necessary to take risks and/or change the course of one's thinking in the decision-making process (Kreuger, 1995).

So, how do you alleviate the fear of having made the wrong decision? One way is to remember that many times decisions are flexible. Kreuger (1995) writes that "most decisions are merely stepping stones to the next decision" (p. 87). Everyone will evaluate your decision from his or her own perspective and position. Thus, you need to be able to justify your decision and be sure your decision reflects your own honest and reasonable viewpoint. Thus, your decision may be affected by your ideals. This is discussed further in the next section of this chapter.

What if one makes the wrong decision? Recall that Butler and Hope (1995) listed "everything depending on making the right decision" as one of the myths related to decision-making. "Often it's the fear of facing that bad choice or of reaching a dead end that keeps people from making decisions" (Kreuger, 1995, p. 88). Thus, by not making a decision, by procrastinating, time may take care of the problem because someone else has made the decision and proceeded without you. Everyone has, at some time or another, made the wrong decision. When this happens, one should just start the decision-making process anew. A careful analysis of the incorrect decision should lead to better questions that can be asked of the involved persons. One can accrue more information that is relevant to the decision-making process.

Kreuger (1995) sums up facing the fear of decision-making with the following statement:

> Whenever you find yourself unable to make a decision or to take action on one you've made, rely on your internal motivator. Verify the soundness of your decision by asking yourself questions. Finally, take action. You need to empower yourself to overcome your fears. Be decisive, and once that decision is made, move into action. (pp. 88–89)

## When Scientific Evidence Does Not Exist to Help with Our Decision-Making

Clinical decision making is based on a reasoned, appropriate decision that is sometimes based on science, and sometimes not! For example, we all have times when we say, "Well, I can't find scientific basis for this decision, but my gut tells me to proceed in this manner." At other times, when involved with a team arriving at a clinical decision, there may be differing opinions. In this case, the decision may be made based on majority rules. A third way is based on our conscience. This implies some tests of ourselves, and requires "thought and insight into the events around us" as we make a clinical decision (Hilton, 1991, p. 21). These three approaches are discussed in depth in the section on Clinical Decision Making. Obviously, we hope there is scientific evidence to back up our decision-making, but this does not always exist, leading to these alternative approaches to clinical decision-making.

Once a decision is made, it is necessary to evaluate the decision in an effort to justify the approach decided on. Hilton (1991) proposes three areas for analyzing the decision: obligations, ideals, and consequences. Obligations may be defined for us by the circumstances and/or people who are either involved in the decision, or affected by the decision in some manner. Hilton proposes that, beyond the legal contract (if it exists), are unspoken obligations that can have an impact on both how the decision is made, and how it is evaluated. These obligations include those associated with friendship, family, profession, trust, and promises. In addition, as health care professionals, we are expected to heal someone and to not extend their suffering.

The second area for analyzing our clinical decisions is ideals. Every health care professional needs to do some self-evaluation to review his or her ideals that may help define and formulate clinical decisions. We are under an obligation to make the best decision for the patient, but there are times when this may conflict with our ideals and personal beliefs. Some examples of ideals upon which there is a general consensus are respect for others, loyalty, justice, truth, and genuinely caring about other individuals (colleagues and patients) with whom we are associating.

Third, one can analyze a decision by evaluating the consequences of the decision. Hilton (1991) proposes the following four questions:

1. What will happen if we take the proposed action?
2. Will it do more good than harm?
3. Will it help more people than it hurts?
4. What would happen if everyone in this situation made the same decision? (p. 21)

Ethicists have varying opinions as to how much consequences should be used to analyze clinical decisions. Hilton proposes that one use consequences as a tie breaker when there are conflicts between two or more ideals and if one has multiple obligations.

## *Making the Decision*

Making the decision for an individual patient will be based on "clinical expertise, the patient's perspective, and the available scientific evidence" (American Speech-Language-Hearing Association, 2008). Reviewing the steps, the SLP first develops the clinical question, searches for and finds the evidence if it exists, and assesses the evidence with regard to its relevance to the patient and the clinical question. All of this does not necessarily reveal an answer, but it may spark an interest in clinically researching the clinicians' instincts when no collaborating evidence exists so that one can be reasonably sure the correct clinical decision has been made.

Butler and Hope (1995) list six strategies that can enhance an individual's ability to make an efficient and effective decision. Their first strategy is called "The Balance Sheet." Some call this a listing of the pros and cons; others list advantages and disadvantages. The problem to be solved should be written at the top of the page, and then the page should be divided into two columns (one pros/advantages, the other one cons/disadvantages).

Their second strategy is to have trial runs and make time projections. Butler and Hope (1995) suggest pretending that a specific decision has been made, then imagining the short and long-term consequences of that particular decision. Then, do the same for the "other side of the coin" going through the same exercise. At the conclusion of these trial runs, ask yourself if the decision feels right, and do you have a "gut feeling" as to which decision is the right one.

Creating a "sounding board" is the third strategy suggested by Butler and Hope (1995). They suggest asking three individuals to listen to your thoughts and "reflect back to you their understanding of your problem and of your inclinations" (p. 389). It is suggested that you do not limit your sounding boards to individuals who are likely to agree with you. Rather, persons who can pose as a "devil's advocate" may be able to introduce some factors for your consideration that you had not thought of previously. Likewise, they may be able to maintain more objectivity than someone to whom you are close or who "thinks like you do."

"Information Gathering and Sifting" is the fourth strategy. Before making decisions, it is "important to clarify the factors which are significant to you, and about which you need more information. Once you know what these factors are, you can think about how to find the necessary information" (Butler & Hope, 1995, p. 390). Once the information is gathered, you can "sift" through the accrued information to evaluate its reliability and accuracy. This is one reason the American Speech-Language-Hearing Association requires graduate practicum and the clinical fellowship year. These experiences give one the opportunity to learn how to gather and sift information related to the provision of services to your patients under the guidance of an individual who has experience in clinical problem solving and decision-making.

Handling chain reactions is a fifth strategy and sometimes the most difficult because it typically affects several individuals. The decisions we make often affect other individuals as well as ourselves. For instance, deciding where to locate a private practice can have implications for the type of clientele who will be able to access your office and for the staff who are driving or using public transportation to get to work.

Finally, Butler and Hope (1995) stress the importance of maintaining one's energy reserves. Do not spend an inappropriate amount of time on a decision. Two factors that interfere with our ability to maintain our energy are fatigue and preoccupation. Fatigue can turn a simple decision into a more difficult one. Preoccupation (sometimes with a major decision) may distract us and make solving the little problems more monumental than it needs to be. When this happens, it is probably a good idea to delegate the decision to someone else, if possible, or put off the decision until you can give it the appropriate amount of attention.

## Critical Pathways

Due to reimbursement and time restrictions often placed on speech-language pathologists who are providing home care, it has become essential that the SLP provide quality care and achieve goals in a shorter amount of time than in the past. In addition, they must provide health care in the most efficient and effective manner possible while focusing on functional outcomes to enhance the quality of life of our patients. In fact, critical pathways provide "documented data and a predictable path of care" (Dikengil, 1998, p. 9) that must be a part of negotiating contracts with managed care organizations.

Dikengil (1998) describes critical pathways as providing "a framework for describing clinical treatment protocols and outcomes that a health care facility expects to deliver to a patient population during a preset number of days" (p. 9). This framework extends from the time treatment begins until the date the treatment ends. Critical pathways provide structure to treatment goals and standardization of the service delivery process by encompassing guidelines for how and when care should be provided. Critical pathways are:

> a framework for coordinating team work, a route to streamlining health care delivery. They are clinical management tools that organize, sequence, and time the major interventions of health care providers. Critical pathways are grounded in CQI (Continuous Quality Improvement) methodology and use its scientific tools, such as teams, flowcharts, data collection, analysis of variance, and so on. A critical path can be thought of as a project management plan. (Shekim, n.d., p. 1)

Critical pathways provide structure to treatment goals and standardization of the service delivery process by encompassing guidelines for how and when care should be provided. As expected, some patients will not conform to the guidelines, so the clinician must be prepared to explain the variance and advocate for increased or different services.

In the 1950s, the concept of Critical Path Method (CPM) came into use as "a tool for project planning in industrial engineering and managerial services" (Shekim, n.d., p. 2). Over the years, CPMs were implemented in a variety of construction, engineering, marketing, and equipment installation businesses. In the middle 1980s, Karen Zander was the first to utilize CPMs in the health care setting as she used the CPM to review the delivery of patient care at the New England Medical Center in Boston, Massachusetts. Also during the 1980s, Congress enacted measures of health care reform ("managed care") in response to the soaring cost of health care, and the call for new methods of managing health care was made. As a result, there was a proliferation of health care agencies, and insurance companies began to dictate who got therapy and how long they got therapy.

Continuous Quality Improvement (CQI) or Total Quality Management (TMQ) was adopted by many health care organizations (providers, purchasers, and insurers alike). CQI, which focuses on processes and systems to improve the efficiency and effectiveness of service delivery, is a methodology designed to improve quality by reducing variance, therefore eliminating inefficiency, rework and waste, and reducing cost. (Shekim, n.d., p. 1)

Critical Pathways attempt to address four core questions:

What is required by each discipline to bring patients with similar diagnoses to realistic outcomes?

What is the best way to produce that work?

Who is accountable for those outcomes?

How can we restructure care so that this happens more consistently? (Dikengil, 1998, p. 9)

To answer these questions, it is suggested that teams be organized to develop and implement critical pathways. For example, a team in a rehabilitation center may consist of a physical therapist, an occupational therapist, the speech-language pathologist, a nurse, a physiatrist, a psychologist, and a social worker. In addition to the professionals on the team, Shekim (n.d.) recommends having former patient(s) and/or their family members as members of the team. After determining the make-up of the team, its team members should list the various disorders that need critical pathways to guide in the provision of efficient, yet effective, treatment. There may be different team members for the various disorders within one setting.

   In this step, if the clinician has determined that the general strategy is inefficient and/or ineffective, he can either (1) change the task or (2) revise the stimulus and response.

## Evidence-Based Practice

According to the American Speech-Language-Hearing Association (ASHA), evidence-based practice (EBP) has a goal of integrating three elements: clinical expertise, best current evidence, and client values in order to reflect "the interests, values, and choices of the individuals we serve" (ASHA, 2004). As defined by ASHA, "evidence-based practice refers to an approach in which current, high quality research evidence services are integrated with practitioner expertise and client preferences and values into the process of making clinical decisions" (ASHA, 2005), the ultimate goal of EBP.

There are four steps in EBP:

1. Framing the clinical question
2. Finding the evidence
3. Assessing the evidence
4. Making the clinical decision (ASHA, 2005, p. 1)

### *Framing the Clinical Question*

To ensure that the evidence will be appropriate for the circumstances faced by the SLP, one has to "frame" the question. ASHA recommends a system known as PICO as an approach to framing the question. PICO is an acronym for population, intervention, comparison, and outcome. They also point out that numerous rewrites may be necessary before the question is in its final form.

"Population" is the description of the clients with a specific disorder. For example, "children with cleft palate" or "patients with dementia." "Intervention" can refer to the type of management (e.g., collaborative or pull-out methods in a school), or specific therapy approaches such as cognitive rehabilitation. "Comparison" would provide a contrasting of different approaches. For example, if the population were stroke patients, the intervention group could be those who get early treatment, and the comparison group would be those who get later treatment. The "Outcome" is what is hoped to be achieved, such as "the child will categorize items according to function," or "the patient will improve his functional communication skills," or the patient with a head injury will be able to resume going to school/work" (ASHA, 2008).

Under the umbrella of evidence-based practice, there are two ruling factors. One is to develop the question based on the clinician's expertise and experiences, then to determine the availability of evidence to support the clinician's decisions. Sometimes research may not be available so that the clinician should either broaden or refine the topic/framed question to take advantage of what is available. Of course, clinicians should always consider doing clinical research and if the clinician has developed an area of expertise in which there is little research available, he or she is obligated to explore the question and look toward publishing his or her plan and outcome (maybe your research will become someone else's evidence!).

## Finding and Assessing the Evidence

Once one has formulated the question to be answered, one begins to search the literature for relevant information that can be used in answering that question. It is always important to take into consideration the "worthiness" and quality of the research being reviewed. Systematic reviews and individual studies can be utilized and assessed when determining whether the information is relevant, reliable, and valid, and if it answers the clinical question posed by the clinician. The credibility of the researchers is another area of consideration, and, in some instances, who funded the research. Pharmaceutical companies are known for funding research on various medications, but when they fund research on their own products they are less likely to report any adverse information that could potentially affect the sales of the products. The design of the research is another factor which should be considered when evaluating the appropriateness and credibility of the evidence (ASHA, 2007).

### *Decision Trees*

Yoder and Kent (1988) edited a book based on decision trees for the assessment and management of over 50 types of disorders related to hearing, speech, and language in adults and children. Their first step in clinical mapping is to identify the communication behavior that needs to be modified. This may include a set of subgoals based on a task analysis of the desired behaviors.

Their second step is to take into consideration environmental factors (patient's daily activities, related behaviors (facilitative or interfering), physical disability, and status of education or vocation as well as personal (goals and self-esteem).

Third, Yoder and Kent advocate the development of a general management goal that becomes the focus of each stage of treatment.

In the fourth step, the clinician(s) "has to identify relevant stimulus and response characteristics" (Yoder & Kent, 1988, p. 1). At this junction, the clinician should also plan where the therapy will take place, how long the therapy will last, and how frequently the patient will be seen for treatment.

An analysis of the components of the therapy may be indicated in the fifth step. It may be necessary to engage in task analysis activities to determine how to best approach the general and specific goals for a given patient.

Finally, the clinician needs to "assess the treatment" if the expected benefits are not being realized. By that, Yoder and Kent (1988) advocate either starting the decision-making process over again, taking care to reevaluate the treatment strategy to determine whether the strategy is a valid one, or revamping the strategy. If it needs revamping, the clinician moves on to the final step.

In this step, if the clinician has determined that the general strategy is inefficient and/or ineffective, he or she can either (1) change the task or (2) revise the stimulus and response.

### *How to Make a Decision*

The key element in the decision-making process is that there must exist a choice (Figure 8-1). If there is only one solution, there is no need for the process because there is no decision to be made. When a choice has been established, one should evaluate each possibility by asking the following four questions (Kreuger, 1995):

1. Does this alternative provide the best solution to the problem?
2. Do we have the resources to implement this alternative should it be chosen?
3. Does this alternative provide the greatest advantage for those involved?
4. Does this alternative create fewer new problems that do the others?

In answering these questions, it may be necessary to use fact analysis and intuition together in order to arrive at a reasonable decision. When defining steps to be used to implement a decision, Kreuger points out that when a decision is made in advance of its implementation, you have some time to judge alternatives in order to be sure you have

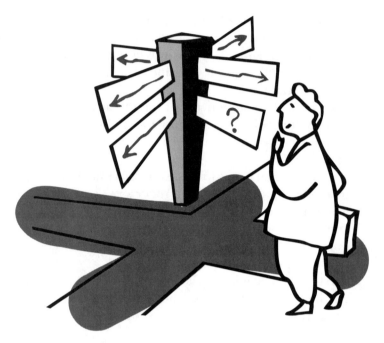

**Figure 8–1.** Often, it is not clear in which direction to go when making decisions.

made the correct decision, and then to "lay the groundwork" for the implementation of the decision.

Schlenger and Roesch (1999) discuss two strategies to be used by individuals faced with making a decision. The first is to set firm deadlines, and they suggest this should include determining your objectives, getting relevant information, clarifying your alternatives, and then making the decision. The second strategy is to create a ranking system. Butler and Hope (1995) also make this suggestion. Butler and Hope advocate assigning a point value to each item on the list in order to give those that are more important more weight in the decision-making process. After assigning a point value to each item, the decision-maker can add up the total number of points and determine which way to proceed in the decision-making process. Schlenger and Roesch take it a step farther, suggesting that each option be listed under things to be done, and then ranked in three ways using a scoring scale of one to five. In addition, Schlengler and Roesch suggest a column indicating whether the task can be delegated. The three areas to be ranked are: (1) importance of job to me, (2) time required, and (3) difficulty. Certainly, similar categories could be determined in your quest to reach a decision, or they can be modified to more closely fit the factors affecting the decision to be made.

Groopman (2007) writes that "working in haste and cutting corners are the quickest routes to cognitive errors" (p. 268). He encourages patients to ask the following questions of their physician when he or she has made a diagnosis with which you are not comfortable. The first question is "What else could it be?" The practice of medicine is not an exact science—there is a realm of uncertainty with almost every decision regarding an initial diagnosis. By asking this question, one can minimize the possibility of an error in thinking such as "premature closure, framing effect, availability from recent experience, and the bias that the hoofbeats are horses and not zebras" (Groopman, 2007, p. 263) by forcing the physician to consider a test or procedure that could further clarify the diagnosis. A second question is "Is there anything that doesn't fit?" which, one hopes, will prompt the physician to consider other possibilities based on the presenting symptoms. The third question proposed by Groopman is, "Is it possible I have more than one problem?" Typically, there is only one problem, but occasionally there may be a multiplicity of anomalies.

> This question is another safeguard against one of the most common cognitive traps that all physicians fall into: search satisfaction. Your question about multiple causes for your problems should trigger the doctor to cast a wider net, to begin to ask questions that he didn't pose before, to order tests that might not have seemed necessary based on his initial impressions. (p. 263)

How do these three questions relate to the diagnosis of a speech, language, and/or hearing problem? Perhaps, as clinicians, we should be asking ourselves these questions prior to making a final decision as to the diagnosis that best fits our patient. Then, in my opinion, we could feel more confident that we have done extensive thinking (both "in the box" and "out of the box") and reached the proper conclusion prior to sharing the information with the patient and/or his or her family. These three questions should minimize haste in our decision-making while leaving the door open for additional input from the patient and/or his or her family.

### Ethical Decision-Making

Sometimes it is difficult to make a decision in light of the Code of Ethics governing one's profession. At times, it may be hard to determine if you really are facing an ethical decision; however, they are more common than we may realize. Typically, an ethical decision involves relationships and responsibilities. There may be competing views from the "other side." There may be a conflict between your values and the rest of the decision-making team. In addition, there are many "gray areas" where no clear-cut answer is available. As you engage in making an ethical decision, you should keep in mind seven questions:

Has something unethical occurred? If so, what? If not, why not?

What are the opposing views?

Who benefits from the situation, and how?

Who does not benefit, and why?

What influences your decision about the situation?
   a) Social parameters
   b) Cultural parameters
   c) Political parameters
   d) Personal beliefs
   e) Previous experience

Once the decision has been made, do you feel it is fair? Why or why not?

What other options could have been considered? (Ducharme, Jodoin, Konieczny, Stanford, Seymour, & Tharpe, 1994)

In 1994, Ducharme, Jodoin, Konieczny, Stanford, Seymour, and Tharpe made a presentation at the annual convention of the American Speech-Language-Hearing Association. They suggested that one participate in a "self-test." This self-test is in Appendix 8A. They also developed an "Ethical Decision Making Worksheet" that is shown in Appendix 8B.

Irwin, Pannbacker, Powell, and Vekovius (2007) developed a schematic (Figure 8–2) for making an ethical decision.

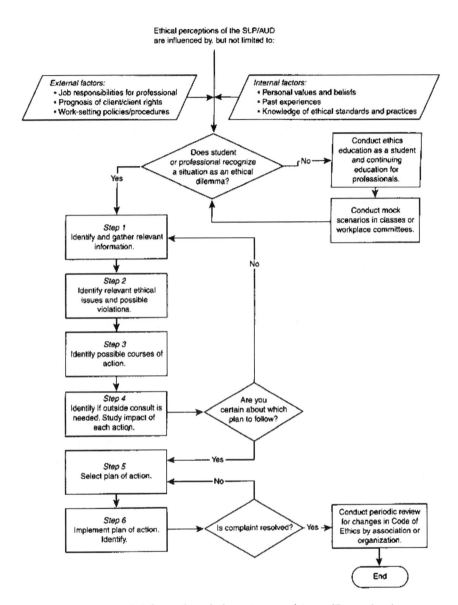

**Figure 8-2.** Model for ethical decision-making. (From Irwin, Pannbacker, Powell, and Vekovius, *Ethics for speech-language pathologists and audiologists: An illustrative casebook*, p. 61. Copyright 2007 Thomson Delmar Learning. Reprinted with permission.

173

## Clinical Decision-Making

As mentioned earlier, in *First Do No Harm*, Bruce Hilton (1991) writes that there are three ways to arrive at a reasoned, appropriate decision: gut feelings, majority rules, and conscience. Conscience implies some tests of ourselves, and requires thought and insight into the events around us. When we analyze a decision, we need to assess our obligations and our ideals. Obligations include legal contracts, obligations of friendship, obligations of family, obligations of our profession, obligations of trust, obligations of promises, and obligation to heal versus our obligations not to extend suffering (as one would possibly find in nutritional issues). When our obligations are in a "tie" with our ideals, Hilton recommends that we use consequences as a tie breaker. Consequences occur in response to three questions:

1. What will happen if we take the proposed action?
2. Will the proposed action do more harm than good?
3. Will the proposed action help more than it will hurt?

Furthermore, sometimes we have to make a choice between competing rights and needs. For example, the debate over the use of fetal tissue implants in patients with Parkinson's disease pits the needs of the patient with the rights of the fetus.

There are also situations in which ethical issues are turned into legislation and/or public policy. (Hilton, 1991, p. 71). For example, in PARC v. Pennsylvania, the parents of children with disabilities filed suit against the state of Pennsylvania saying that children with mental handicaps were entitled to a free public education. This case laid the foundation for the Education for All Handicapped Children Act of 1975, making the decision on education of children with handicaps a matter of public policy and legislation, not personal wishes, ethics, and beliefs.

### *Factors That Can Interfere With Effective Decision-Making*

Butler and Hope (1995) list nine "pitfalls" that can create havoc with the decision-making process. These are as follows:

1. **Biased thinking**

2. **Categorical thinking** ("There's only one right answer or one completely wrong answer"): One can avoid categorical thinking by asking him/herself the following questions: "How could you live with the choice you have made, what adaptations will it demand of you, whether it is a permanent choice, and whether it could be changed if things work out differently from the way you expected?" (p. 392)

3. **Not thinking beyond the decision:** Things are constantly changing. Try to anticipate changes that could occur that potentially would have an effect on the decision.

4. **Conservatism:** There is a certain degree of comfort in thinking about maintaining the status quo, but we often do not learn by doing so. I once attended a conference where several participants wore circular buttons that said "TTWWADI" with a red line drawn through it (as in the "No Smoking" signs). The letters stood for "That's The Way We've Always Done It" and, of course, the red line said that is not the way to achieve anything.

5. **Confusing problem solving with worrying:** Individuals need to acknowledge that some decisions are bigger than others. Some decisions require more time to think through than others, and some people think they always should be able to solve a problem quickly. When a quick, well-considered decision is not made, they may start to worry about it, which, in turn, can make the decision more difficult.

6. **Information tangles:** Butler and Hope (1995) maintain that misinterpreting information and forgetting information are two of the biggest negators to the process of decision-making. They suggest "keeping a notebook, using information sources efficiently, and asking others to keep you up to date" (p. 392). A decision cannot be a good one if it is made without all the necessary information.

7. **Expect the feeling to come first and the decision to follow:** This belief can stall decision-making. Usually, when a tough decision has to be made, one will feel better after it is made than while waiting to make the decision.

8. **Fears and worries:** Some decisions can make life a bit uncomfortable. Butler and Hope give the example of a person who accepts "a promotion that involves speaking in front of large groups" when the individual has a fear of public speaking. It may be helpful to involve more than one person in making a major decision that could impact not only yourself, but the welfare of others as well.

9. **Other "bad" feelings:** Stressors (e.g., finances) and distressers (e.g., fatigue) can interfere with decision-making. Sometimes factors need to be "put on hold" until a decision is made. If there are stressors and distressors in an individual's life, it makes sense to postpone the decision or involve others in the decision.

## Is Your Decision the Right One?

Kreuger (1995) proposes the following questions to help you decide if the decision you have made is the correct one:

1. How good is the information I have gathered and interpreted?
2. What objective do I intend my decision to achieve, and what will happen if the objective is not achieved?
3. Once the decision has been made, how is it executed? What is your plan of action?
4. What can go wrong during the execution of the decision?
5. What further decisions will be necessary as a result of the first?

By using these questions, one can carefully analyze the decision that has been made, and proceed with the implementation phase with confidence that the correct decision has been made.

## Summary

Schlenger and Roesch (1999) label ineffective decision-makers "Fence Sitters" and characterize them as individuals who frequently worry excessively about small decisions and become paralyzed when faced with making a major decision. They suggest the following tips in order to make a reasoned decision:

1. Learn to evaluate your needs and desires.
2. Realize that in most situations, there really are no wrong choices. Any outcome, good or bad, will give you feedback that you can use to improve your decision-making abilities.

3. Break down your decisions into a series of small steps with individual deadlines.
4. Pinpoint your fears so that you can deal with them directly.
5. Use a ranking system when comparing a number of different alternatives.
6. Get input from a knowledgeable friend.
7. Pay attention to your instincts—your gut feeling.
8. Take time to relax and reward yourself along the way (pp. 105–106).

These tips sum up the different ideas offered in this chapter. The reader should develop his or her own systematic approach to problem solving based on the discussion in this chapter. No one system is going to work for everyone, so several alternative approaches to problem solving were presented in hopes that the reader can find a system of decision-making that works well for him or her.

# References

American Speech-Language-Hearing Association. (1993). *Ethics: Resources for professional preparation and practice.* Rockville, MD: Author.

American Speech-Language-Hearing Association. (2004). *Report of the joint coordinating committee on evidence-based practice.* Rockville Pike, MD: Author.

American Speech-Language-Hearing Association. (2005). *Evidence-based practice in communication disorders* [Position statement]. Available from: www.asha.org/policy

American Speech-Language-Hearing Association. (2008). *Evidence-based practice.* Retrieved from: www.asha.org/members/ebp/

Butler, G., & Hope, T. (1995). *Managing your mind: The mental fitness guide.* New York: Oxford University Press.

Dikengil, A. T. (1998) *Handbook of home health care for the SLP.* San Diego, CA: Singular.

Ducharme, Jodoin, Konieczny, Stanford, Seymour, & Tharpe. (1994, November). *Ethical decision-making: Do the right thing.* Presented at 1994 Convention of the American Speech-Language-Hearing Association. New Orleans, LA.

Groopman, J. (2007). *How doctors think.* New York: Houghton-Mifflin.

Hilton, B. (1991). *First do no harm: Wrestling with the new medicine'slife and death dilemmas.* Nashville, TN: Abingdon Press.

Irwin, D., Pannbacker, M., Powell, T. W., & Vekovius, G. T. (2007). *Ethics for speech-language pathologists and audiologists: An illustrative casebook.* Clifton Park, NY: Delmar Thomson Learning.

Kreuger, C. (1995). *Hit the ground running: Communicate your way to business success.* St. Paul, MN: Brighton.

Schlenger, S., & Roesch, R. (1999). *How to be organized in spite of yourself: Time and space management that works with your personal style.* New York: Signet.

Shekim, L. (n.d.). *Critical pathways.* Rockville, MD: American Speech-Language-Hearing Association.

Yoder, D. E., & Kent, R. D. (1988). *Decision making in speech-language pathology.* Philadelphia: B. C. Decker.

## APPENDIX 8A
### Self Test*

A. For statements 1 through 6, indicate whether you strongly disagree, disagree, are neutral, agree, or strongly agree.

1. Right or wrong depends on the situation.
2. Sometimes it is OK to break the rules.
3. Most successful professionals set their principles aside at one time or another.
4. Women are more ethical than men.
5. Most speech-language pathologists and audiologists are honest.
6. Ethics are absolute principles.

B. How do you feel when you observe unethical behavior in your classes/clinic? (Circle all that apply.)

1. Confront the person, but do not report it.
2. Do nothing about the situation.
3. Report it to superiors.
4. Report it to superiors anonymously.
5. Other (Specify) _____

C. Which of the following kinds of ethical violations have you observed in your classes/clinic?

1. Bribery
2. Cheating on exams/papers
3. Discrimination
4. Favoritism/nepotism
5. Lying to peers/supervisors
6. Sexual harassment
7. Violations of confidentiality

D. For each of the following student situations, indicate if you observed it (yes or no), and whether you consider it not to be a violation (1), to be a minor violation (2), or a major violation (3).

1. You see students cheating on an exam.
2. You hear fellow student clinicians loudly discussing particular clients. They are mentioning the names and details of the case.

---

*From "Ethical Decision Making: Do the Right Thing" presented at ASHA, 1994 by Ducharme, Jodoin, Konieczny, Stanford, Seymour, and Tharpe

3. A student clinician accepts a gift from a client.
4. You have received an assignment to collect data on language development in a kindergarten class. When you get there, the teacher introduces you to some parents as a speech-language pathologist from the university, and you do not correct her.
5. A graduate clinician becomes emotionally involved with one of his/her clients.

E. For each of the following professional situations, indicate if you observed it (yes or no), and whether you consider it not to be a violation (1), to be a minor violation (2), or a major violation (3).

1. An SLP diagnoses a child's problem based solely on the mother's description.
2. An SLP/Audiologist becomes emotionally involved with one of his/her clients.
3. You work at an exclusive private clinic. One day you walk into the bathroom and see your colleagues smoking marijuana.
4. You are invited to a private party where you see your colleagues using illegal drugs.
5. An SLP is instructed to treat a laryngectomee even though he or she has never worked with this population.
6. A fellow professional is making sexual advances toward other clinicians.
7. A colleague recommends treatment whose effect on a particular client is questionable.
8. A public school SLP is pressured by a child's parents to provide therapy that she believes is unnecessary.
9. An audiologist recommends a suitable hearing aid to his or her clients. The manufacturer has promised a bonus for each of the hearing aids that he or she sells.
10. An SLP is running a tight schedule and reduces her therapy sessions with a client from one hour to 45 minutes. However, in order to get reimbursed, the clinician continues to state in her reports that the sessions are an hour long.
11. A clinician counsels a client who has depression that stems from a communication disorder.

## APPENDIX 8B
## Model for Ethical Decision Making Worksheet*

1. Do you think something unethical occurred? If so, what; if not, why not?

2. What are opposing view coming out of this situation?

3. Who benefits from the situation that has occurred: How? Who does not benefit: Why?

4. What influences your decision about the situation? Discuss any items below that also influenced your decision:
   a. social parameters
   b. cultural parameters
   c. political parameters
   d. personal beliefs
   e. previous experience

5. Once a decision/choice is made, do I/we feel it is fair? Why?

6. What other recommendations/choices could have been made to resolve the dilemma?

---

*From From "Ethical Decision Making: Do the Right Thing" presented at ASHA, 1994 by Ducharme et al., 1994.

## APPENDIX 8C
## Ethical Decision Making

### I. COMPONENTS OF AN ETHICAL DILEMMA
A. May be hard to determine if you are really facing an ethical decision.
B. Are more common than we realize
C. Involves relationships and responsibilities
D. May have competing views from "the other side"
E. May have competing values
F. Will face many "gray areas"

### II. HOW DOES ONE MAKE AN ETHICAL DECISION?
A. Has something unethical occurred?
B. What are the opposing views?
C. Who benefits from the situation, and how?
D. Who does not benefit, and why?
E. What influences your decision about the situation?
F. Once the decision is made, do you feel it is fair?
G. What other options could have been considered?

### III. ETHICS CALIBRATION QUICK TEST
A. What was violated?
B. Who appears to benefit the most? In whose best interest is the decision, anyway?
C. How will the decision make me feel about myself?
D. Whose evidence is most convincing?
E. What values are in conflict?

---

*Note:* Appendix 8C is partially an expansion of an ASHA Ethics Resource, and partially an expansion on the work of unknown authors.

*Chapter 9*

# Goal Setting:
# Setting and Achieving
# Life Goals

*We tend to* let *things happen* to *us, when we should be* making *things happen* for *us."*

Waitley (1996)

Goal setting is an approach to personal organization and exploration that many of us neglect to do. However, if one defines a mission statement, and then lists what he or she will do to fulfill this mission, he or she is well on the way to improving life in all settings and roles. Furthermore, when setting one's goals, one should be focused on the results, not the activities (Covey, 2004). It may be necessary to have one set of goals for work, one for home, and one for socialization.

Covey (2004) (Figure 9-1) writes the following:

> Roles and goals give structure and organized direction to your personal mission. If you don't yet have a personal mission statement, it's a good place to begin. Just identifying the various areas of your life and the two or three important results you feel you should accomplish in each area to move ahead gives you an overall perspective of your life and a sense of direction. (p. 137)

Heller (1999) suggests that tasks one faces can be divided into four categories: very important, important, useful, and unimportant. This should be combined with "time elements: urgent (to be done as

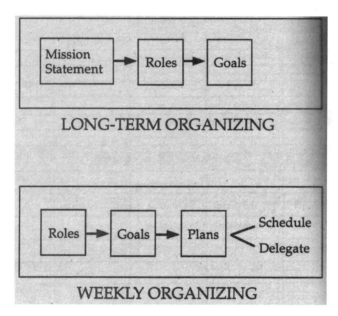

**Figure 9–1.** Long-term and weekly organizing chart. (From S. R. Covey, *The 7 habits of highly effective people* (p. 168). Copyright 2004 Free Press. Reprinted with permission.)

soon as possible), fairly urgent (to be done by a near deadline), not urgent (can wait for a while), and optional (no time pressure)" (p. 44). This helps to organize one's goals and priorities.

Denis Waitley (1996) coined the term "Flextactic" meaning to "make flexibility the key to your success" (p. 1). Flexibility will often require that you change your personal paradigms, which includes learning to be as comfortable with the unfamiliar and unknown as you are with the familiar. A paradigm is "a pattern or set of guidelines that influences the way you look at your life" (Waitley, p. 1). Occasionally, one runs into obstacles that can be a source of frustration, or a new way of looking at a situation. Waitley (p. 2) proposes the following questions that one should ask when faced with an obstacle:

1. Did I cause this obstacle by my own actions or lack of them?
2. Did someone else cause this obstacle?
3. Is this obstacle one that grew out of the natural progression of circumstances?

Davidson (2004) writes that one should organize his or her activities of life as a way of determining one's goals. The first step is to write down things that are important to you. This includes items that are assigned to you by someone else and that you plan to achieve. These become your goals. After taking a break for several hours, Davidson suggests that one review the list to see if any items can be deleted or combined. Too many goals/priorities can lead to frustration and anxious feelings. After the first review, "restructure, redefine, and rewrite your list" (p. 38). Repeat this process again, making final revisions on the priorities. After this last review, make a working list of those items that are a priority and set out a timeline for meeting them.

## Thermodynamics and Goal Setting

As taught in high school physics, the first law of thermodynamics states that "the amount of energy in a closed system always remains constant. In other words, the energy put into a system must always be balanced by energy going out" (p. 5). Waitley (1996) suggests that the concept of thermodynamics can be applied to helping one achieve his or her goal by saying that small energy consumption is needed to achieve small goals whereas valued or important goals demand more effort and energy. Thus, it is helpful to break down major goals into smaller subgoals that can be more easily achieved. In addition, subgoals can be adjusted when necessary and are easier to change than large goals.

## Rules for Achieving One's Goals

Waitley (1996, pp. 9–13) proposes four rules to help one achieve his or her goals:

*Rule One:* Believe in Your Dreams and Goals

As positive energy, belief is the promise that hoped-for goals will at last be realized. As negative energy it's the premonition of our deepest fears and unseen feelings of inadequacy. (p. 9)

*Rule Two:* Clearly Define Your Goals

Successful people formulate achievable goals and action plans. In defining clearly stated goals, one can develop a "sense of direction" to facilitate the achievement of his or her goals. As part of defining one's goals and dreams, one should "project dreams and goals into definitive periods of time, and set their own target dates for achievement." (p. 10)

*Rule Three:* Do What It Takes to Win

Successful people are willing to put time, energy and effort into making their plans work. Perseverance is a key to meeting goals.

*Rule Four:* Remain Adaptable to Change

Sometimes reality knocks at our door harboring the need to make changes. Change is inevitable and requires that one be adaptable and flexible. Change should be viewed as an opportunity to learn, and possibly to develop a different, but often better, path to attaining one's current and future goals. Waitley writes that envisioning the future "requires both imagination and a clear view of reality." (p. 13)

As a side note, the author suggests that this quote serves as an excellent guide for therapy as well as for personal goal setting!

## Evaluate Your Motivators

The best motivation is an inner, intrinsic force "that inspires you to solve a problem, fill a need, or do something truly excellent" (Waitley, 1996, p. 21). However, we can be equally motivated through extrinsic motivators such as a paycheck. Waitley (1996) has identified six forces that can motivate people to achievement:

1. "Status with authority figures: Doing something to gain the respect of experts or supervisors.
2. "Status with peers: Doing something so that others will look up to you.
3. "Acquisitiveness: Wanting to own something so much that you'll do anything to get it.
4. "Competitiveness: Desiring to do something so that you can do it bigger and better than anyone else
5. "Concern for excellence: Constantly working at something to make it the best it can possibly be

6. "Achievement via independence: Mastering something for the sake of having the freedom to do it on your own terms" (p. 22).

Freedom and flexibility, not bureaucracy, are operative words in achieving one's goals. When one defines needs in his or her life, these needs can become the harbinger of a goal. The intensity of the need coupled with "determination, optimism, and toughness" (the DOT principle) (Waitley, 1996, p. 28) will dictate how motivated one is to achieve that goal. Determination, optimism, and toughness all have stamina as a key component. "Determination gives you the resolve to keep going in spite of the roadblocks that lie before you" (p. 28). Determination is partially defined by "stamina," which Waitley (1996) describes as "the strength to withstand disease, fatigue, and hardship. It includes a sense of purpose, steadfastness, and a commitment to solve problems" (p. 29).

He also states that "stamina includes an outgoing, warm temperament," (p. 28) which is a key component of optimism. Being optimistic helps one focus on the attainment of his or her goals and helps provide the energy to keep one from getting in a rut and seeing setbacks as insurmountable.

"Toughness gives you the resilience to keep pressing on, even if your determination and optimism are lagging" (p. 28). With regard to toughness, if one has stamina he or she has the flexibility to adapt to change while standing up to any chaos that occurs as the result of changes.

An additional strategy to achieve one's goals is to visualize the completed goal. (Davidson, 2004). One way to do this is to shut the door on routine activities and allow yourself to ponder on the goals and how your life will be more organized and in control. Then, notes to oneself should be placed near sites one can easily see at home, in social settings, and at work.

## In Search of Self-Definition

Waitley lists four basic questions one should ask him- or herself when searching for self-definition:

1. If it weren't for time, and personal responsibilities, what would I really love to do with my life? In other words, if I were free to

do whatever I wanted, what would I be doing tomorrow morning (p. 32).

2. What did you love to do as a child? What were you really good at? What made you feel proud?
3. What makes you feel that way now?
4. Are you doing something to benefit other people? Does that give you a feeling of self-respect and fulfillment? (p. 33)

**Task Block 1:** Take Waitley's four basic questions above and answer them for yourself.

In the process of defining one's self, focus plus flexibility are required. On the one hand, one needs to stay focused among myriad distracters. On the other hand, one needs flexibility to handle unexpected alterations to the plan for achieving one's goals. Waitley (1996) suggests that one should write life-forming, self-defining goals, then organize them by dividing the goals into those that are long-term (those that take more than three years to accomplish), intermediate (six months to three years to complete), and immediate goals (those that can be achieved within three to six months). Immediate goals can be further broken down into small, attainable steps.

## Flextactics

Waitley (1996) coined the term "flextactics" as a set of guidelines for setting and achieving one's personal goals. The components are as follows:

Learn to Thrive on Risk

Make Your Life an Open Book

Use the Power of Visualization

Create a Blueprint for Success

Turn Obstacles into Opportunities

### *Learn to Thrive on Risk*

Achieving one's goals often requires that one have a healthy acceptance of risk, which is a key ingredient for achievement.

There are a number of ways to take risks based on one's personal risk-taking style. For example, do you learn from previous mistakes and move forward, or do you let the mistakes become an insurmountable obstacle to achieving your goals? If one focuses on the long shot, he or she does not "master the step-by-step building process that leads to lasting achievement" (Waitley, 1996, p. 15).

Flextactics encourages one to be a risk taker, and to learn from the past and implement that knowledge in planning your future. Set goals that are "flexible enough to survive the constantly changing environment we live in" (Waitley, p. 31).

## Make Your Life an Open Book

Although many of us keep a journal depicting events and significant people in our lives, some of us use a journal as a means of setting our personal goals in life and following a path to their fruition. Waitley (1996) advises that the first entry should be based on recognizing your "greatest character strengths. Second, identify your natural talents and abilities" (p. 41). Based on the results of steps one and two, one should make a notation of education, volunteer, and job experiences that have enhanced or created new information related to one's knowledge and skills. Finally, one should take note of personal and professional acquaintances who can serve as a sounding board and offer constructive feedback, and of those who have influence and can assist in networking with persons of similar interests and abilities.

## Use the Power of Visualization

The whole purpose of goal setting is based on an ability to visualize your goals. Waitley (1996) writes that "this can dramatically enhance your motivation for making those goals come true" (p. 51). This helps individuals to keep the long-term goals in focus while simultaneously achieving smaller goals.

Exercises to stimulate creative imagination include forming mental images to help remember and benefit from other individuals' input. In addition, visualizing your goals will help achieve your goals and increase your enthusiasm for doing so.

Visualize the person you want to become five and ten years from now. Waitley (1996) encourages us to plan a day based on our projected goals, then do the same for ten years hence. The purpose of visualization "is to help you 'see' all the unlimited opportunities that are (y)ours for the taking" (p. 59).

### Create a Blueprint for Success

Review your life-forming goals. "Then, beside each one, list all the benefits you'll gain when the goals have been achieved. Be detailed, be vivid, and make the benefits real for you. Keep in mind the importance of concentrating or focusing your energy" (p. 63). This will enable you to prioritize your goals. Davidson (2004) suggests that any goal one sets for him or herself be written down, quantified, and given a deadline to achieve the goal. Once prioritized, do a "reality check." If "you can formulate a practical plan consisting of manageable steps in order to reach a given objective," the goal is realistic (p. 64). Ask yourself these questions during the process:

a.  "Are you in a position of responsibility for your own achievement? Does success or failure depend primarily on you?" (p. 64)
b.  "Having taken responsibility for your own success, do you still take into account the help you'll need from others?" (p. 66)
c.  "Have you examined your individual goals in terms of importance and difficulty of attainment?" (p. 67)
d.  "Do any of your goals require you to act in a way that's completely out of step with your temperament and character?" (p. 68)
e.  "Is the time frame you envision for goal achievement both challenging and realistic?" (p. 68)
f.  "Have you considered the obstacles that you may encounter, and have you devised ways to turn them to your advantage?" (p. 70)

### Turn Obstacles into Opportunities

As part of a self-analysis, identify weaknesses and/or deficiencies related to one's objectives, noting "5 things about yourself that you believe you need to strengthen to reach your goals in the allotted time" (p. 75). Waitley (1996) refers to the deficiencies are part of a "Personal Inventory Postscript." Next, one needs to analyze his or her strengths, knowledge, and skills and then determine which ones can be used to bolster and/or eliminate the deficiencies. It is helpful to make a checklist of obstacles which Waitley defines in the following way:

> The obstacles that you see blocking your way are really, for the most part, your own learned perceptions. They are misinformed prejudices against yourself, and prejudice limits vision. Prejudice keeps you focused on what you *think* exists, rather than what *can* and *should* exist. Prejudice stifles creativity and prevents problem solving. (p. 77)

### *Flex-Planning Ideas*

Some other ideas to remember include:

1. "Schedule longer, uninterrupted blocks of time for special projects" (p. 78).
2. "Prepare for delays and plan for interruptions" (p. 78).
3. "Ask yourself, 'If I knew I had exactly twenty years left to live, what would I do differently in terms of goal setting and priorities?'" (p. 79)
4. "Even with all the steps mapped out, you must be able to readjust your goals" (p. 79).
5. "If your first plan fails . . . regroup and try again!" (p. 79)
6. "We tend to *let* things happen *to* us when we should be *making* things happen *for* us" (p. 81).

### Summary

Davidson (2004) writes that one must take charge of his or her own goals, and personalize those goals that are put upon you by others. He suggests that one ask the following questions before starting to work on one's goals:

1. What will be involved?
2. What kind of energy will you lend to the assignment?
3. What will you do first?

4. How will you take charge?
5. How will you feel when the task is completed? (p. 46)

These questions allow one to take ownership of his/her priorities and goals in life. It is hard work to achieve one's goals, but Waitley (1996) writes seven principles that make hard work hard but enjoyable:

1. "Think of your work as a challenge, not a chore" (p. 97).
2. "Approach whatever you are doing as if it were your first time" (p. 97).
3. "Follow the 'as if' principle. When you must do work that is dull and repetitious, do it as if it were interesting" (p. 98).
4. Keep track of your progress toward your goals and take pride in your accomplishments (p. 98). "Don't wait for somebody else to encourage your efforts and to show appreciation for your work. Take pride in your own work on a daily basis" (p. 99).
5. "Keep the end result in sight" (p. 100).
6. "Set up a dynamic daily routine" (p. 100).
7. "Schedule time for relaxation and exercise" (p. 102).

If one adopts the principles and procedures outlined in this chapter, one will be more organized, and will focus on goals that enable you to complete the items you have determined to be a priority.

## References

Covey, S. R. (2004). *The 7 habits of highly effective people.* New York: Free Press.

Davidson, J. (2004). *The 60 second organizer.* Avon, MA: Adams Media.

Heller, R. (1999). *Achieving excellence.* New York: DK.

Waitley, D. (1996). *The new dynamics of goal setting: Flextactics for a fast-changing future.* New York: William Morrow.

# Chapter 10

# Counseling Patients and Caregivers Living with a Communication Disorder

*If you are to make a difference in your helping relationships with others, it means helping others to change their lives in such a way as to make the consequence of their living more satisfying."*

H. Hackney and S. Nye (1973)

## Introduction

Two key ingredients to being a successful speech-language pathologist are knowing how to be a patient-oriented clinician and ensuring that clients are educated about their disabilities or handicaps, or both. Dikengil (1998) writes that "counseling is an integral part of providing rehabilitation to the communication impaired patient and his or her family. By understanding the nature of loss, the grieving process, and patient's beliefs, the speech-language pathologist may be able to offer appropriate counseling" (p. 63).

Spremulli (1997) outlined several guidelines to follow in being sure that effective client education is provided. The first guideline is to outline what to expect in therapy. In the postassessment conference, the clinician reviews the tests that were administered and interprets the results for the client and/or caregivers, or both. As part of this process, the clinician should explain how this information along with information gained from the history, the family interview(s), and your clinical observations will be used to develop goals and procedures that will be addressed in therapy. Discussion about the effectiveness of therapy in similar cases can take place, but under no circumstances should a clinician make any promises about the outcome of therapy. Numerous variables affect the results of treatment; this needs to be explained to the client and caregivers so that they have no false expectations that could lead to dashed hopes.

The second guideline is to gain knowledge of the client's views and expectations. Questions asked at this time should focus on exploring how the disability affects the individual and his or her family. Understanding what the clients and caregivers expect as a result of therapy also is important information. Exploring these topics can provide the clinician with some degree of understanding as to how realistic clients are in their acceptance and knowledge of the disability.

The answers to these questions also can help establish an understanding of the client's knowledge about his or her disease or disorder. Clients and their caregivers arrive for therapy at different levels of awareness. Some have spent time researching the disorder, contacting support groups, and learning all they can from a variety of sources. Others rely on the speech-language pathologist to provide them with some of this initial information. Thus, the clinician should be knowledgeable about the disorder and its typical impact on communication.

Once the clinician has an appreciation of the client's and caregiver's views, expectations, and knowledge, he or she should focus the initial therapeutic efforts on empowering the client and his or her significant others to be part of the therapeutic process. That is to say, the clinician must maximize the client's ability to participate in and carry out the therapy (Spremulli, 1997). One of the best ways to encourage a client's motivation to succeed in therapy is through the active involvement of the client and his or her significant others in therapy planning. This can be done through mutual participation in setting the goals for therapy and keeping lines of communication open between the clinician, the client, and the caregivers.

The clinician must understand the disease or disorder in the broad context of the client's entire life. In acquired disorders, the clinician should learn about the client's life prior to the onset of the communication deficit. An adult patient who has aphasia is likely to feel confused, anxious, afraid, embarrassed, and frustrated as a result of the effect of the aphasia on receptive and expressive language. Feelings of stupidity also are common. Thus, it is critical that the clinician acknowledge that the current status of the patient's speech and language skills does not reflect his or her communication skills prior to the onset of aphasia. To understand this, the clinician must spend time with the patient and/or his or her caregivers exploring the patient's interests, vocation, and avocations prior to the onset of the problem.

The clinician needs to distinguish between disability and handicap. Most of the people that speech-language pathologists see have a developmental problem, an illness, or an injury that affects their ability to communicate. However, the ability to cope with the impairment or disability varies from person to person. The social and personal effects of the disability create the handicap. Many patients' have severe disabilities (a defect, disorderπ, or disease), but are minimally handicapped. Others may have a mild disability, but a severe handicap because they allow the disability to control their actions and beliefs. It is the degree of severity of the handicap, not the disability, that frequently has the strongest impact on the level of patient compliance and satisfaction with the therapeutic process.

## Patient Satisfaction

Keeping the patient satisfied is a key element in having him or her participate actively in the therapy process. Client satisfaction can be defined as the degree to which the patient's beliefs and expectations are met (Spremulli, 1997). To maintain a level of patient satisfaction, it is the clinician's job to be sure that the patient's expectations match reality. Achieving a reasonable and realistic level of expectations is partially dependent on timing. At a time when a patient or family members are dealing with the illness or injury that resulted in the communication deficit, the clinician is asking them to embrace a new way of learning. At the same time, the patient is expected to "understand, integrate, and implement new or different ways of doing things" (Spremulli, 1997).

The clinician who buys into the belief that an educated patient is a satisfied patient has to understand that clinical education is more than the exchange of information regarding the illness and treatment plans. Spremulli (1997) writes that the crucial element in patient education is not the exchange of information but the examination of the nature of the patient's expectations about the respective roles and responsibilities. This reflects the concept of empowering the patient and family members to be key players in the therapeutic process. Simply possessing accurate information about the cause and effects of the disorder is only weakly related to the eventual outcome, particularly in cases in which the cause is a chronic disease process. Rather, the clinician's understanding of the patient's expectations is the more powerful element in effective treatment.

The second critical element in effective therapy is patient compliance. Spremullli (1997) defines patience compliance as "the extent that patients are obedient and follow directions." Sometimes, despite the clinician's best efforts, patient compliance is low. In part, this may be due to a poor conceptual understanding of the goals as a result of the language deficits. Patients may be unclear about the roles and expectations of themselves, the clinician, and the family members. Emotional concerns and issues often interfere with the patients' and caregivers' abilities to receive, process, and recall the information provided by the clinician. Thus, it may be necessary for clinicians to repeat critical information several times in the initial stages of treatment. The patient's ability to accept this information depends in large part on his or her level of awareness of the communication deficit.

The emotional components can dominate a person's view of him or herself and interfere with participation in therapy. In this case, the speech-language pathologist needs to refer the patient/family member(s) to an appropriate person (i.e, psychologist, psychiatrist, or mental health counselor) to resolve the emotional aspects after which they can return to therapy.

## Counseling

There are many different definitions of counseling and different opinions as to what activities constitute counseling. The word *counselor* encompasses a range of practices from psychoanalysis to financial counseling. Mental health counselors, geriatric counselors, vocational counselors, and employment counselors are only a few of the types of counselors (Stewart, 1986). Thus, it becomes imperative to define counseling as it relates to speech-language pathology. Counseling in the health care professions has many purposes: to share information, to offer guidance when asked, to assist a patient or family members in understanding the impairment, disability or handicap, to offer encouragement when a therapy task is difficult, and to listen when appropriate and necessary. Pre- and postassessment interviewing may be part of the process, although the interview itself does not constitute a counseling relationship. Although the definitions of counseling are numerous, a unifying theme is helping an individual to facilitate goal setting and to create change in response to a problem or adversity. These goals and changes are based on a person's academic knowledge of the situation, his or her behavioral response to the adversity it presents, and the person's value and belief system that helps define his or her response to daily situations.

Stewart (1986) addressed the definition of counseling in relation to helping parents of exceptional children. According to Stewart, two critical processes must occur in the relationship with the parents: learning and acceptance. Through learning about the disabilities, a change in behavior that is a necessary element in reaching a satisfactory solution occurs. When clients acquire, develop, and utilize effective and appropriate coping skills, their self-confidence increases. Through increased learning and self-acceptance, the parents become more fully functioning and able to maintain a family life while assisting their child with a disability in realizing his or her fullest potential. Although these statements are aimed at the counseling of parents, they certainly hold true for the counseling of children and spouses of adults who experience an illness or injury that threatens their communication abilities.

## Information Counseling

Patients and families dealing with a newly diagnosed disability are faced with learning about the disability and its impact on their lives. In the early time periods after the onset of the disability, much information is provided by a series of professionals. The problem is that most patients and caregivers are not ready to receive and process information because they are still in the throes of accepting the changes and altering their expectations. Providing too much information before the patient and family members are ready to hear it can add to their sense of confusion (Luterman, 1996). Luterman describes the following approach to information counseling:

> As professionals, we have a responsibility to provide information. As a general rule of thumb, I do not give clients information unless they ask for it. I generally ask, "What do you need to know?" When I receive a response such as "I don't even know enough to ask a question," which is fairly typical in the early stages, one might respond, "It sounds like you are pretty confused." This is an invitation to talk about client feelings. I have seen professionals who are anxious to get things going tell parents who are too confused to ask questions, "Here are some things I think you need to know." This response must be resisted at all costs because it takes away client power and gives the professional too much responsibility. The content questions will emerge as the clients become more comfortable with their new status and are moved a bit further along in the grief process. If we facilitate the process by empathetic listening, the content will emerge. (Luterman, 1996, pp. 61–62)

When the patient or caregiver is ready to receive more information, he or she will ask. At that time, clinicians should answer their questions using a minimal amount of professional jargon. The purpose of providing information is to answer questions, not to overly impress someone with the use of words that are meaningless to most patients. Also, if the clinician offers an opinion when answering a question, it should be qualified as such. The clinician must differentiate between fact and opinion. It is also acceptable for the clinician to tell a client when he or he is "stumped." It is better to admit to not knowing an answer (but offering to find the answer) than to guess incorrectly, thereby providing wrong information.

## Levels of Awareness

### Minimal Awareness

Initially, patients and caregivers are at a level of minimal awareness; they are still at the point of refusing to recognize the abnormalities. They frequently look for other, often unfounded, causes to explain the symptoms. They also believe that the problem will resolve in a short period of time, with or without treatment (Stewart, 1986).

## Partial Awareness

Clients and caregivers who are partially aware of the client's problems begin to describe symptoms to the clinician and often will ask the clinician questions about the etiology of the problem. Typically, these individuals will hope for improvement, but they have a nagging fear that it will not happen. Thus, they begin to question their ability to cope. As a professional, the clinician feels that the patient and/or caregivers have some awareness of the true problem, but they are not ready emotionally or academically to accept all the implications and ramifications of the disorder (Stewart, 1986).

## Considerable Awareness

With time, patients and caregivers reach a level of considerable awareness of the problem and its implications. At this stage, they recognize the disability and its potential influence. They also understand that treatment will help, but there are limitations to how much recovery to expect. At this level of awareness on the part of the patient and caregivers, the clinician should anticipate requests for information about the appropriate treatment and expectations (Stewart, 1986). Thus, this is the time when the patient and caregivers are ready to accept their roles in the therapeutic process. Even though the clinician has stressed the empowerment of the patient and family members from the time of the first session, it is not until the level of complete awareness is reached that they are ready to assume their assigned roles. With this readiness to face the task at hand comes an acceptance of the situation.

# The Grief Process

Just as it is important to determine the patient's and caregiver's level of awareness, it also is crucial to determine where they are in the grief process. Crowe (1997, p. 31) writes that, "if experienced normally, grief is a beneficial process wherein individuals work their way through various emotions to positive acceptance of distressing circumstances." Long accepted as a series of steps related to the acceptance of the death of a loved one, the grief process also plays a role in the acceptance of a disability. The individual who has an acquired disability must mourn the loss of his or her "old self"—the person he or she was prior to the onset of the disorder. The family, too, must mourn the death of the person as they have known him or her and come to accept the "new" person who has been redefined by the illness or injury.

The grieving process lets the client "buy time to find the inner strength needed to deal with" the loss (McFarlane, Fujiki, & Brinton, 1984, p. 7). As grieving is a natural and necessary process, it makes sense that the grieving individual needs acceptance, not judgment, as he or she experiences the components of the grief process. Clients need to know that it is all right to have the emotions they are experiencing. If clients "are allowed to share these feelings without being patronized or judged, most will eventually emerge capable of dealing with the problem. However, if such feelings are repressed, this emergence may be significantly delayed" (McFarlane et al., 1984, p. 7).

Mandell and Fiscus (1981) adapted the grief stages established by Kubler-Ross in 1969 based on her observations of terminally ill patients and their families. Again, although the adaptation was designed to describe the stages through which parents of disabled children progress, these stages and their descriptions also can be used to delineate the stages that patients and families undergo when faced with a communication disorder, regardless of the age or the nature of the disorder.

### *Denial*

The first stage is denial. Denial is actually a primitive and normal response employed by individuals in an attempt to reject a frightful and painful reality. During this stage, the family and patient refuse to believe that the disability exists. Alternatively, they may acknowledge that it exists but minimize its impact and deny that it is a reason for concern (Crowe, 1997). Because they do not believe that the disability actually exists, it is impossible for those in the denial stage to realize the impact of the communication disorder on the entire family (Mandell & Fiscus, 1981). This stage of the grief process corresponds with the minimal level of awareness. It is important that the clinician not confuse overt optimism with denial, particularly when the patient and family members are in the early stages of dealing with the disability.

Kubler-Ross (1969) identified three factors that might influence the existence and recalcitrance of denial in grieving:

1. The accuracy and completeness of information about the illness or disorder determine if and for how long an individual will express denial. If accurate and full insight emerge only after considerable time, denial also might also extend over time and acceptance be delayed.

2. The time an individual needs to resolve grief might affect duration and intensity of denial. A patient facing imminent death has only a short time to work through the grief stages, so he may be feeling the pressure of time and the need to come to terms with fate before confronting it. Others may see the inevitability of fate with so much dread that they become fixated in denial, or any, stage of grief. On the other hand, those who are experiencing a long-term illness or disability may not feel they are in any hurry to come out of denial. Others with long-term problems may very quickly decide that the problems are real, that they are not going to go away, but that they intend to lead productive lives regardless of the impairment. These individuals are anxious to work through the grief and proceed with therapy.

3. An individual's premorbid tendency to rely on denial as a defense against life's pressures increases the probability and intensity of its presence with illness or disability. If a client used denial as a buffer against bad news prior to the onset of the communication disorder, he is likely to stay in the denial stage longer after the onset. In fact, for many of these individuals, denial is the most prominent stage of the grief process.

Patients who are in denial are not good candidates for therapy. The denial process interferes with the ability of both the patient and family members to concentrate on the matters at hand. Thus, much information that is shared with a family in denial will need to be repeated and reinforced at a later time. Also, the patient will have difficulty concentrating on the tasks in therapy. Until the denial can be resolved, the patient is not likely to see any purpose in participating in therapy. Therefore, benefit from therapy will be minimal.

### Guilt

The second stage of mourning is the guilt stage. Mandell and Fiscus (1981) described three forms of guilt. The first form, and the least common one, is attributing the deficit to something that happened in the past. For example, the mother of a disabled child may blame the child's condition on two aspirin tablets she took prior to finding out she was pregnant. In most cases, these past events actually have little or no impact on the existence of the disability. A second form of guilt is described by the statement, "Bad things happen to bad people, therefore, I am bad." In this case, the patient or family member believes that he or she caused the condition to occur in some way. A communication disability is a "bad thing" that requires tremendous adaptations for an individual. Believing oneself to be a bad person will have a negative effect on a patient's self-esteem and self-concept. This negative effect, in turn, may lead a patient to believe that he or she should not get better and thus may interfere with the therapeutic process. The third form of guilt, and the most frequently seen, is the belief that the impairment is punishment for something the patient has done. For example, if a husband and wife quarrel, and the husband has a stroke shortly after the quarrel, the wife may believe that the stroke is punishment for the quarrel.

### Depression

The third stage of the grief process is depression. Mandell and Fiscus (1981) defined depression as "anger turned inward." In this case, the family members and the patients become depressed because they are unable to make the disability go away. In many ways, depression signals the beginning of acceptance because the patient and family realize that the patient's problems are not going to disappear magically and that the disorder they are facing is now part of their lives (Crowe, 1997). This is a critical stage because individuals who have chronic or deep depression should be referred to a psychologist or psychiatrist for counseling that goes beyond that which the speech-language pathologist should provide. It may even be necessary to suspend therapy until the person is able to work through his or her depression.

Depression can be a good or bad sign. As a good sign, it heralds the arrival of acceptance. However, if it becomes self-perpetuating, it can become a major barrier to progress in therapy (Crowe, 1997).

Kubler-Ross (1969) distinguishes between two types of depression:

1. Reactive depression: This is a reaction to the associated events of the loss. It may include reactions over the cost of hospital care and pharmaceuticals, isolation, and the loss of attractiveness. The client with reactive depression may exaggerate the significance of the loss.
2. Preparatory depression: Preparatory depression occurs in terminally ill clients who are preparing for their final separation from this world. Attempts to cheer up the client with preparatory depression devalue the significance of the loss.

In Crowe's book, Wohlman (1989) notes that "depression is differentiated from terms such as sadness, unhappiness, and sorrow because depression, unlike those emotions, involves feelings of helplessness, and a personal sense of guilt for being helpless" (Crowe, 1997, p. 38). The client who has depression may give up on therapy and lose hope for improvement. A downward emotional spiral can be created when the client assumes self-blame that leads to a loss of self-esteem. The loss of self-esteem may lead to increased guilt which, in turn, deepens the sense of depression. The client who is in the throes of depression will make little progress in therapy. An individual with severe depression should be referred to a psychologist or psychiatrist for further treatment.

Crowe (1997) points out that depression is the reverse feeling of anger. The individual who is angry becomes aggressive toward all those who are perceived to be involved with his loss. However, the person with depression becomes passive, although there may be an increase in anxiety, with the development of obsessive behaviors and thoughts. How long the depression lasts may depend on the actual disabling potential of the loss, and the client's perceptions of difference, disorder, or handicap. Because an organic loss has a poorer prognosis, depression may last longer in those cases than in those with a functional loss. Finally, the prognosis for correction or compensation for the loss also affects the duration of the depression stage.

## *Anger*

Anger is the fourth stage of the grief process. Anger can be expressed as "Why me?" or it can remain unspoken. Unfortunately, unspoken anger can lead to a resentment, and even hatred, for the individual with the disability (Mandell & Fiscus, 1981). It is not unusual to see a vacillation between depression and anger, or between anger and guilt, because a family member feels guilty for being angry at the person with the disability, particularly if it is a child. When the patient is angry at him or herself, it is not unusual to see the anger manifest itself as low self-esteem with or without depression. The same type of anger can occur in spouses or adult children because they cannot make the condition go away to make life better for the disabled family member (Luterman, 1996).

The individual in the anger stage may resent the clinician and caregivers, and may be a difficult individual with whom to deal. Anger may be misdirected at the clinician, but the clinician needs to remember that the anger is a consequence of the loss, and not a reaction to intervention (Tanner, 1999). The degree of anger may depend, to some degree, on the potential for the diagnosis to be disabling and/or handicapping, and on the prognosis. Individuals who have an organic etiology may feel more anger because of the potential for the diagnosis to be more debilitating. There may be secondary crises associated with the diagnosis, including role reversal, financial problems, job-related consequences, mental health problems, relationship issues, and self-concept issues (Crowe, 1997).

Clinicians should be aware of this stage of the grief process because they may bear the brunt of the patient's (or family member's) anger. The clinician's job is to make the patient better and to gain the trust of the family. If the expectations of the patient and family are that the patient can be cured by the clinician, they will be angry at him or her if this does not happen. This is why it is crucial to empower the family as part of the diagnostic and therapeutic processes. Each family member, including the patient, should have a role to play. This empowerment and assigning of roles will help prevent anger due to unfulfilled expectations.

The clinician can also bear the brunt of displaced anger. Displaced anger occurs when the patient is angry at him or herself, but takes it out on another individual. This also happens with caregivers who may be angry at the patient for having the disability but take this anger out on other family members or the speech-language pathologist. In both instances, the anger is the result of unmet expectations; the patient expects the clinician to make his or her problems go away, and the family expects the patient to make the problems disappear.

To help the client cope with his or her anger, the clinician should remain nonjudgmental and offer strong, consistent reinforcement of the client's attempts to achieve his or her goals in therapy. Continued counseling can help the client examine and express his anger and channel it in productive directions. Strong support from family members and significant others is critical in extending the comfort of therapy into the client's natural environments. Early success in therapy can also help to abate the anger (Crowe, 1997).

## *Bargaining*

Mandell and Fiscus (1981) introduced a stage they call bargaining into the grief process. In this stage, the family members or patient, or both, make a "last ditch" attempt to make the disability go away. That is, they make a final effort to change the existing circumstances and return to their predisability life. Often, these bargains take on a religious or altruistic theme. For example, the patient may promise to never miss another Sunday in church if God will make the disability disappear.

## *Acceptance*

The final stage is acceptance of the impairment, disability, or handicap. Once the client reaches the stage of acceptance, he or she no longer needs to expend energy on the psychological resolution of the loss, and can channel all energies toward rehabilitation (Tanner, 1999). "Acceptance symbolizes a client's conscious awareness of the reality that he or she is and may always be a person with a communicative disorder until an earnest attempt is made to do something about it" (Crowe, 1997, p. 39). Acceptance symbolizes resolution of the loss and an acceptance of the situation (but not necessarily its limits) (Tanner, 1999). The person who is in the acceptance stage has considerable awareness of the circumstances. He or she is ready to be empowered by the clinician to be a part of the therapeutic process in order to regain the maximum ability possible. Tanner (1980) points out that acceptance and resignation should not be confused. Resignation implies acceptance of one's fate without hope of resolving the disorder; the client feels helpless about creating any change in the future. Acceptance is an acknowledgment of the person's fate, but without the feeling of helplessness. The resigned patient will not be a good candidate for therapy until he or she is willing to take some responsibility for improving the situation.

Crowe (1997) also points out the need to differentiate between resignation and acceptance. Resignation indicates that the individual has accepted his or her fate and feels helpless to do anything about the future. Acceptance, on the other hand, is the result of acknowledgment of the realities of one's fate. We can help clients remain at a level of acceptance by explaining to them, carefully and in detail, evaluation results, prognosis, and therapy procedures and rationales. However, the clinician should remain vigilant to the client's level of motivation and not assume that, because the client has reached the level of acceptance, motivation is no longer a concern.

Stages of grief imply that the grief process is a lock-step sequence of emotions and events. First, it is important to recognize that people progress through the grief process at varying rates. For example, one gentleman who had been diagnosed as having amyotrophic lateral sclerosis (Lou Gehrig's disease) progressed through the grief stages in a matter of hours. Another family took almost two years to work through the stages of grief after the birth of a child with disabilities. Second, not everyone will pass through every stage. Furthermore, the clinician should not assume that, once a stage is passed, that the individual will not return to a previous stage. This happens frequently when a family's firstborn is disabled and the second child is nondisabled. Before the birth of the second child, the parents would become quite excited about the strides made in therapy. However, after watching the second child master the progression of speech and language skills without extensive therapeutic intervention, the parents sometimes regress to the depression and anger stages of the grief process and must work through those emotions again. Thus, there is a fluidity to the grief process. It is not always measured in finite steps that, once passed, are never revisited.

The clinician's interaction with the grieving client can significantly impact the client's ultimate acceptance of the impairment, and also affect his or her motivation and desire for intervention. It is critical that the clinician understand the grief process because interruption of the process can reduce the client's motivation for therapy. It can also interfere with the client-clinician relationship. Short- and long-term goals can be altered and/or postponed when the grief process is interrupted. The interference can also lead to the maintenance of counter-productive measures (Tanner, 1980).

## Counseling Interviews

A counseling interview is one that is used to influence someone's attitudes and/or behaviors. It provides both release and support for the interviewee(s). In a counseling interview, the clinician should provide the client, family members, and/or caregivers with support and direction, and encourage them to express their feelings and attitudes about their difficulties (Shipley, 1992). This is also the time to "modify their methods of interaction, to assist in the treatment, or to understand and correct the ways they may be hindering the client's progress" (Shipley, 1992, p. 10).

Depending on the length of time between the onset of the disorder and the information-giving interview, the client and/or his or her family members may express a variety of emotions. These include anger caused by fear, a feeling of being threatened, and frustration. There may be an underlying sense of vulnerability, pain, and anxiety. The interviewees may express defensive reactions, of which there are six types:

1. Reaction formation: The client and/or family members immerse themselves in activities in order to appear supportive and hide the resentment;
2. Suppression: The client and/or family members keep their true feelings to themselves;
3. Repression: Consciously, for this person, the problem is nonexistent, therefore it does not need to be addressed;
4. Rationalization: The individual using rationalization focuses on the positive actions that need to be accomplished and forgets the actions that did not get it done, because he will continue to rationalize about what has not gotten done;
5. Displacement: The person using displacement may express anger by slamming doors or creating scapegoats;
6. Projection: Through projection, the client and/or his or her family members transfer blame, excuse failures, and minimize their own weaknesses (Shipley, 1992).

## Effective Listening

To counsel patients and their families through the stages of the grief process, the clinician must master the skill of effective listening. Barbara (1958) listed four critical factors that determine the effectiveness of a person's listening: (1) concentration, (2) active participation, (3) comprehension, and (4) objectivity.

### *Concentration*

Concentration requires the listener to remove any distractions from the immediate environment. For example, if the counseling session is being held in the clinician's office, telephone calls should be placed on hold and a note should be placed on the door advising others not to interrupt. Concentration also requires patience (Shipley, 1992). Owing to the nature of the communication disorder, a patient may offer numerous tangential comments. The clinician needs to guide the patient artfully back to the topic of concern, and this guidance has to be patient and nonabrupt. Likewise, family members may need this time to acquaint the clinician with the patient's life as a person prior to the communication disorder. In the case of parents with a young disabled child, this may be a time when the parents talk about their nondisabled child or their hopes and expectations for the child before he or she was born. There are many responses that a clinician can offer to a grieving patient or family member. It is important for the clinician to pay close attention, even during these periods of "rambling," and not let other concerns and thoughts interfere with the listening process.

### *Active Participation*

A counseling clinician needs to remain alert during the counseling process and be ready to offer information or guidance when it is requested.

One of the least helpful statements is one that is often offered in sympathy: "I'm sure things are not as bad as they seem." For the patient or family member, things *are* as bad as they seem. Offering a denying response interferes with the patient's and family's ability to face the seriousness of their situation. The use of close-ended questions (yes-no answers) also is an ineffective listening activity. In fact, it is better to use reflective statements that paraphrase what the patient or caregiver has said than it is to ask questions. When it is necessary to ask questions, they should be open-ended to facilitate the exchange of more information. The most effective means of actively participating in the exchange of information in a counseling situation is to listen for the feelings and thoughts that the patient expresses. Learning to rephrase the feelings and thoughts expressed by the patient and/or caregiver is one of the most effective listening devices the clinician can use.

## Comprehension

When listening for comprehension, the clinician not only listens to the surface expressions but also listens for the meanings that underlie the spoken messages. The clinician conveys that the message has been received by remaining somewhat detached throughout the process (Shipley, 1992). This is not to say that the clinician is cold and uncaring. In this case, "detached" refers to the ability of the clinician to remain objective yet actively involved in understanding what the speaker is trying to convey.

## Objectivity

When listening objectively, the clinician avoids imposing his or her personal attitudes, beliefs, and feelings on the patient or family members. When opinions are expressed, they should be identified as such. The clinician uses reflective listening to help maintain objectivity. If the clinician poses a question, he or she should be prepared to explain the rationale behind the request. Some questions may be personal, so the clinician must be able to justify any question that is asked. In fact, the clinician should carefully consider all questions that he or she plans to ask. If there is no use for the answer, the question should not be asked.

## *Active Listening*

The term *active listening* implies that the message receiver and the message sender are integrally involved in the exchange process. The challenge in counseling is to keep the patient or caregivers talking so that the maximum amount of information is obtained in the least amount of time. By using active listening skills, this can be accomplished. A key to effective listening is to decipher what the patient or caregiver is feeling and what the message means. The clinician then puts this understanding into his or her own words and feeds it back to the patient or family member for verification. Usually, the clinician does not send a message of his or her own but only reflects what the patient or family member is saying back to the sender of the message.

## The Role of the Speech-Language Pathologist

Counseling by the speech-language pathologist is appropriate when it is part of a holistic approach. Self-reliant clinicians and clients focus on the present and on those changes that can be made now in the pursuit of personal growth. Growth can only occur when the client feels the control and power of the present and challenges a perceived negative or stagnant self-image. Although the clinician may employ counseling techniques in the treatment of any communication disorder, it is particularly important in the treatment of voice and fluency disorders, and in the treatment of clients with lifelong and/or life-threatening illnesses, such as ALS and cancer. Care must be taken during the cognitive stages of therapy not to make the client too dependent on the clinician-client relationship in order to succeed. Another problem that affects generalization and maintenance is when the client is struggling with disabling emotions; that is, he may be getting more out of being disabled than being healed.

It is important that the client's self-concept be addressed throughout therapy. The clinician must take into account the questions, "Is my client's self-concept altered by the presence or absence of the communication disorder?" Do the disabling emotions continue even after the communication disorder is resolved? Therapy should address the cognitive and affective components of the client's self-concept. Clients should be taught that it takes less personal strength to support coping behaviors than to support defensive, resigning, and/or withdrawing behaviors. Occasionally, the speech-language pathologist may be faced with a client who has a psychogenic communication disorder. In these cases, it is necessary to demonstrate didactically that therapy is not needed. It is important to address the clients' fears and concerns, and not to dismiss their concerns too quickly. This is because the perceived disorders are very real to clients. It may become necessary to refer these clients for further professional help from a psychiatrist or psychologist (Vinson, 2001).

### Sympathy and Empathy

One of the biggest mistakes a clinician can make when participating in counseling activities is to offer sympathy. Sympathy is defined in *Webster's New World Dictionary* (p. 1356) as a "sameness of feeling; affinity between persons or of one person for another" (Guralnik, 1970). It is further defined as "an entering into, or the ability to enter into, another person's mental state, feelings, emotions, etc., especially pity or compassion felt for another's trouble, suffering, etc." The job of the clinician is not to reach a homeostatic level with patients and family members. No matter what the clinician may think, it is not possible to understand "what it feels like" to be in their shoes. Even if a family member of the clinician's underwent a similar loss of communication abilities, he or she cannot possibly know what it feels like to that family. This is because of the myriad individual factors that affect how well a family faces an illness or injury that alters the expectations and realities that family has for its family members. In fact, offering a sympathetic statement such as, "I know how you feel" can generate a defensive remark from the patient and family members as they exclaim that no one can possibly know how they feel. In addition, trying to reassure a family member sympathetically that "things are not as bad as they seem" denies them of the right to temporarily feel self-grief and self-pity, which are, in the long run, important aspects of the acceptance process.

Although it is counterproductive to offer sympathy, clinicians can offer a level of empathy. In the same dictionary, empathy is defined as "the ability to share in another's emotions or feelings" (Guralnik, 1970, p. 407). Empathy entails trying to understand the feelings of another person so that these feelings can be validated, not minimized as they are when sympathy is offered. In this case, the clinician acts as a willing and active listener for the patient and/or family members. The clinician's use of effective listening skills helps the individuals involved to express to the clinician the degree to which the disability is affecting them. It does not set up a defensive reaction because the clinician is not trying to assume or downplay their hurt and confusion. Rather, the clinician is trying to serve as a sounding board against which the family can measure its level of readiness and awareness.

When a person offers empathy, the message is "I understand." When an individual offers sympathy, the message is, "I feel sorry for you." Unspoken, but still implied, in the sympathetic message is the message that the clinician is somehow superior to the person to whom the illness, injury, disability, or handicap has occurred because the problem has happened to the other person (Stewart, 1986). Empathy, therefore, is a tool that can be used to determine the nature and depth of the patient's or family member's concerns and to establish a counseling relationship with the individuals in need.

## *Intellectual Support*

A second major job of the speech-language pathologist is to provide intellectual support on how to establish a facilitative environment. The level of interaction between the client and clinician should be analyzed for its appropriateness. The clinician should determine if the family members are using a language level that is too simple, or too sophisticated, for the patient. He or she should also be sure that attempts at communication have not ceased as a result of frustration with the communication process. A patient who is constantly misunderstood may stop making the effort to communicate. Likewise, if the patient expresses frustration at being misunderstood, the caregivers may give up trying to understand the patient and, with time, a mutual expectation that no communication efforts will be made arises. Thus, one of the jobs of the speech-language pathologist is to explore different means of interacting with the patient to facilitate communication efforts. This may include trying augmentative or alternative communication devices such as sign language, gestures, or communication boards (ranging from simple picture boards to elaborate communicators with digitized or synthesized speech).

## Referrals

A third role of the speech-language pathologist is to make appropriate referrals when necessary. As alluded to earlier, it may be necessary to refer the patient and/or caregivers for counseling in dealing with the adversity they face. If the patient seems "stuck" in the partial awareness level or appears unable to work through to the acceptance stage of the grief process, additional counseling beyond that within the speech-language pathologist's scope of practice may be needed.

### Offer a Reasonable Overview of the Future

Another major responsibility of the speech-language pathologist is to provide a reasonable overview of future expectations. This will assist the family in making long-term plans, which include financial considerations as well as emotional and physical factors. In the case of a patient with Alzheimer's disease, the clinician should explain the progression of the disease and help the family plan for respite care if and when it becomes necessary. If a family is dealing with the birth of a disabled child, the clinician can help explain the educational opportunities that are legally mandated for the child. It will always be helpful, regardless of the disorder or age of the patient, to put the families in contact with local support groups that can provide assistance beyond the limits of what the speech-language pathologist can provide.

The most important role of the speech-language pathologist is to follow through on empowering the family to act together to define the goals and develop programs to reach those goals. In the empowering process, the clinician should not be afraid to share his or her own weaknesses and doubts. It is also acceptable, and desirable, to admit when he or she is stumped and make any referrals necessary to help the family stay active in the rehabilitation process.

## Summary

Speech-language pathologists often find themselves in positions that require some knowledge of counseling and an appreciation of the role that counseling plays in establishing a relationship with a patient and his or her caregivers. Initially, the counseling may be in the intake interview when the clinician is finding out more about the patient as the evaluative process begins. However, the role as a counseling clinician expands during the sharing of information that follows the initial testing of the patient. As the clinician empowers the patient and family members to be part of the therapeutic process, this role expands even further. The speech-language pathologist should be aware of the level of awareness of the patient and the caregivers as well as where they are in accepting the communication deficit. Understanding the patient's knowledge of the communication disorder and the readiness of the patient and family members to accept the disorder and make the necessary adjustments can greatly enhance the therapeutic process.

To be effective, the clinician must want to hear what the patient and family members have to say and genuinely want to be helpful. The clinician must be able to accept the opinions and feelings offered by the patient and his or her family and trust them to work through their feelings to find workable solutions.

A communication disorder can alter a patient's self-concept, so it is critical for the clinician to determine the role a disorder plays in defining the patient's self-concept. The main goal of the counseling process is to have the patient's perceptions match the external reality so that he or she will have realistic expectations for therapy. The clinician strives to create an environment in which the patient takes charge of his life, instead of having the communication disorder control his or her existence (Crowe, 1997). The goal is not to think as one person but to understand as two individuals on a team working toward the maximum capabilities possible.

According to ASHA, the expected outcome of counseling is

> to develop appropriate goals for recovery from, adjustment to, or prevention of a communication or related disorder by facilitating change and growth in which patients/clients become more autonomous, more self-directing, and more responsible for achieving their potential and realizing their goals to communicate more effectively. (ASHA, 1993, p. 19)

# References

American Speech-Language-Hearing Association. (1993). Preferred practice patterns for the professions of speech-language pathology and audiology. *Asha, 35*(Suppl. 11), 19–20.

Barbara, D. A. (1958). *The art of listening*. Springfield, IL: Charles C. Thomas.

Crowe, T. A. (1997). *Applications of counseling in speech-language pathology and audiology*. Baltimore: Williams & Wilkins.

Dikengil, A. T. (1998). *Handbook of home health care for the speech-language pathologist*. San Diego, CA: Singular.

Guralnik, D. B. (Ed.). (1970). *Webster's New World Dictionary of the American language* (2nd college ed.). New York: World.

Hackney, H., & Nye, S. (1973). *Counseling strategies and objectives*. Englewood Cliffs, NJ: Prentice-Hall.

Kubler-Ross, E. (1969). *On death and dying*. New York: Macmillan.

Luterman, D. M. (1996). *Counseling persons with communication disorders and their families* (3rd ed.). Austin, TX: Pro-Ed.

Mandell, C. J., & Fiscus, E. (1981). *Understanding exceptional people*. St. Paul, MN: West.

McFarlane, S. C., Fujiki, M., & Brinton, B. (1984). *Coping with communicative handicaps: Resources for the practicing clinician*. San Diego, CA: College-Hill Press.

Shipley, K. (1992). *Interviewing and counseling in communicative disorders: Principles and procedures*. New York: Merrill.

Spremulli, M. (February 17, 1997). Is our patient education effective? *Advance*.

Stewart, J. G. (1986). *Counseling parents of exceptional children* (2nd ed.). Columbus, OH: Charles E. Merrill.

Tanner, D. C. (1980). Loss and grief: Implications for the speech-language pathologist and audiologist. *Asha, 22*, 916–928.

Tanner, D. C. (1999). *The family guide to surviving stroke and communication disorders*. Boston: Allyn & Bacon.

Vinson, B. P. (2001). *Essentials for speech-language pathologists*. San Diego, CA: Singular.

Wohlman, B. B. (1989). *Dictionary of behavioral science* (2nd ed.) New York: Academic Press.

# Chapter 11

# The Supervisory Process

## Introduction

Being a supervisor of student clinicians, paraprofessionals, or other professionals in and out of the field (for example, being a rehabilitation director) is thrust upon most of us at one time or another. However, it is probably one of the roles for which we are least prepared; supervision is a process that is typically learned "on the job." The purpose of this chapter is to provide an overview of this process and whet the appetite of supervisors to do further reading in this dimension of their jobs. By way of introducing the topic, Appendix 11A is a Supervisor/ Supervisee's Bill of Rights as developed by ASHA (1977).

## The Purpose and Dimensions of Supervision

Casey, Smith, and Ulrich (1988) state that the purpose of supervision is "to prepare professionally competent individuals who are capable of self-analyzing, self-evaluating, and independent problem solving" (p. 5) Supervision has an interpersonal dimension and an analytical dimension.

The interpersonal dimension of supervision involves the interactions of the supervisor and supervisees. Many of the same interaction qualities found between clinician and patient can also be found in the interactions between supervisors and their charges. For example, rapport is a critical component of any client/clinician relationship.

Likewise, it is a critical component between supervisors and supervisees. In Table 11-1, the author writes that the word "rapport" can be an acronym denoting the interactions between these two groups of individuals.

Cogan (1973) also stressed the importance of the supervisee/supervisor relationship being based on colleagueship as opposed to one of superior-subordinate relationships. This basis leads to joint problem-solving, and emphasizes the value of each player in the supervisory process. Valuing the role each player has in the supervisory process is underscored in the Competencies for Effective Clinical Supervision (see Appendix 11B).

**Table 11-1.** Elements of Rapport (RAPPORT)

| |
|---|
| **Respect:** to hold in mutual regard the roles the supervisor and supervisee play in their interactions |
| **Admiration:** to hold in esteem the supervisees' efforts to improve his or her clinical knowledge and skills; for the supervisee to appreciate the role the supervisor plays in his or her own professional development |
| **Participation:** to develop a learning program that empowers the supervisee and the supervisor to be active participants in the supervisee's learning |
| **Professional Interaction:** to maintain a professional, yet personal, level of interaction between the supervisor and supervisee. |
| **Opportunity:** to go with the flow and take advantage of situations that present themselves in accordance with the supervisee's need to learn |
| **Restraint:** for the supervisor to become less directive and more accommodating of the supervisee's learning efforts, thereby encouraging active participation and encouragement of the supervisee in his or her own knowledge and skills acquisition |
| **Timing:** to be cognizant of a supervisee's readiness to receive and accept information and suggestions from the supervisor |

*Source:* Adapted from *Language Disorders Across the Lifespan* by B. Vinson. Copyright 2007 by Thomson-Delmar Learning.

## *An Analytical Dimension*

The analytical dimension of supervision is what gives meaning to the objective data accrued through the observation activity. McCrea and Brasseur (2003) write that in the analysis aspect of supervision,

> The data are examined, categorized, and interpreted in relation to the change, or lack of change, in the client or clinician. Analysis comes naturally from the planning and observation stages because if planning is well done, both supervisor and supervisee will have determined exactly what data will be collected and what will be done with them. (p. 39)

Glatthorn (1984) defined clinical supervision as being a systematic and carefully designed process to assist students in their professional development. The process typically involves a preconference in which the student and supervisor meet to determine the focus of the impending observation, and discuss the content of the session. The supervisor then watches the session and collects pertinent data. This is followed by the supervisor's analyzing the data gathered in the observation, then meeting with the supervisee. (This process is similar to the clinical process of analyzing a client's language and speech skills through the diagnostic process.)

## Supervision as a Collaborative and Cyclical Endeavor

Supervision is "collaborative" in the sense that it includes participation and problem-solving by the supervisor and clinician. Most graduate students and beginning assistants have had little if any experience instructing people with communication disorders. They must learn about the nature of the disorders they encounter as well as the means for assisting the clients in overcoming their disorders. This early stage requires direct assistance from the supervisor. As the supervisee gains experience, the focus of the supervision should include the supervisee's becoming increasingly independent of the supervisor. Dowling (2001) summarized the work of Cogan (1973) in stating that the cycle of supervision that "begins with establishing the relationship between the supervisor and supervisee and is followed by planning, observing, collecting data, analyzing and conferencing, and then returning once again to the planning stage" (p. 31).

## Five Components of the Supervisory Process

Based on the work of Goldhammer in 1969, Jean Anderson developed five components of supervision that are specific to the field of communication sciences and disorders. As cited by Casey, Smith, and Ulrich, Brasseur (1987) and Anderson (1988) elaborated on each of the five components by listing the tasks associated with each component.

1. **Understanding** the Supervisory Process:
   a. The components of the supervisory process
   b. Supervisee's perceptions about supervision
   c. Goals and expectations for supervision
   d. Prior experiences in supervision
   e. Styles of supervision and supervisee preferences
   f. Supervisee anxieties
   g. Needs and competencies of the supervisee for placement on the continuum of supervision (p. 14).

2. **Planning:** Determine and prioritize objectives for the clinical (clinician and client) and supervisory (clinician and supervisor) interactions:
   a. What will be observed, that is, the specific data to be collected
   b. How the observation will be accomplished (methodology)
   c. How the observational data will be analyzed
   d. How the analyzed data will be interpreted (criteria)
   e. How the findings will be integrated (future planning) (Casey, Smith, & Ulrich, 1988, p. 18)

3. **Observing:** The observation component is the one in which the supervisor objectively watches the supervisee. It is critical that supervisors who are observing maintain objectivity, not subjectivity. Just as a clinician would keep data on the performance of a client in therapy, the supervisor needs to keep data on the supervisee's skills and abilities. This will set up a stage for the fourth component of the supervisory concept.

4. **Analyzing:** In the analysis stage, the supervisor logically interprets the objective data and observations. The tasks associated with this stage include the examination, categorization, summarization, and organization of raw data, and the consideration of the data in relation to specific objectives.

5. **Integrating:** The supervisor and supervisee share results of the analysis and mutually agree on the conclusions. This is best accomplished in a "problem-solving conference." (Casey, Smith, & Ulrich, 1988)

## Tasks of Supervision

In the position statement by ASHA, *Clinical Supervision in Speech-Language Pathology and Audiology* (1985), there is a list of 13 tasks of supervision. These tasks are listed in Table 11–2.

For purposes of discussion, some of the tasks have been combined in the following explanations of the tasks.

1. Establishing and maintaining an effective working relationship with the supervisee: As clinicians, we see the importance of having a good working relationship with our clients, with "good working relationship" defined as having mutual respect, shared goals, and good rapport. The same is true of the relationship between the supervisee and the supervisor. Early on in the process, the goals for the supervisee need to be identified, and then the supervisor and supervisee should work as a team to ensure that those goals are met.

2. Assisting the supervisee in developing clinical goals and objectives: We set goals for clients by analyzing their strengths and weaknesses based on observation, spontaneous speech/language samples, and standardized testing. There is not a standardized test one can give a supervisee to see what his or her clinical skills are, so observation and frank conversation between the supervisor and supervisee serve as the basis for determining the goals and objectives for the supervisee.

3. Assisting the supervisee in developing and refining assessment skills and clinic management skills: Quite obviously, these two areas will dominate the professional life of a majority of speech-language pathologists so they must be a focus in the supervision process. There are a variety of methods one can use to provide supervision of students and clinical fellows who are studying to hone the assessment and treatment of individuals with speech/language/swallowing/hearing disorders.

4. Demonstrating for and participating with the supervisee in the clinical process: Demonstration therapy is a key element in the

**Table 11–2.** ASHA's 13 Tasks of Supervision

| |
|---|
| 1. Establishing and maintaining an effective working relationship with the supervisee |
| 2. Assisting the supervisee in developing clinical goals and objectives |
| 3. Assisting the supervisee in developing and refining assessment skills |
| 4. Assisting the supervisee in developing and refining management skills |
| 5. Demonstrating for and participating with the supervisee in the clinical process |
| 6. Assisting the supervisee in observing and analyzing assessment and treatment sessions |
| 7. Assisting the supervisee in development and maintenance of clinical and supervisory records. |
| 8. Interacting with the supervisee in planning, executing, and analyzing supervisory conferences. |
| 9. Assisting the supervisee in evaluation of clinical performance |
| 10. Assisting the supervisee in developing skills of verbal reporting, writing, and editing. |
| 11. Sharing information regarding ethical, legal, regulatory, and reimbursement aspects of the profession. |
| 12. Modeling and facilitating professional conduct |
| 13. Demonstrating research skills in the clinical or supervisory processes |

*Source:* From *Position Statement on Clinical Supervision in Speech-Language Pathology and Audiology.* Copyright American Speech-Language-Hearing Association, 1985. Reprinted with permission.

supervision process. Some students can grasp the essentials of interaction with clients without much demonstration while others will require repeated examples of "watching the pro" do the clinical tasks. The same prompting hierarchy (Figure 11–1) that is

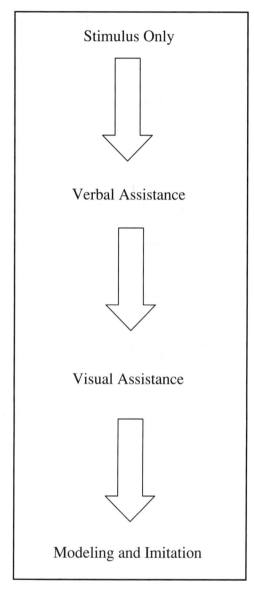

**Figure 11-1.** Prompting Hierarchy

applied in a clinical setting with clients can be used to guide the supervisee along the path of achievement of skills associated with the clinical process.

The supervisor provides the stimulus (instructional directions) to evoke the desired response from the supervisee. If the supervisee is unable to respond appropriately, the supervisor can offer verbal assistance as a clue to the desired response. If that is ineffective, the supervisor can provide visual assistance such as drawing a chart or graph to demonstrate how to document a patient's progress. On the prompting hierarchy, the next prompt should include the supervisor's modeling of the desired response, and the supervisee, in turn, would imitate the desired response.

5. Assisting the supervisee in observing and analyzing assessment and treatment sessions: In the opinion of the author, one of the most difficult tasks we undertake is teaching students and clinical fellows how to analyze and interpret test results and data collected in treatment sessions. The ability to analyze and interpret this information is best taught to a supervisee by guiding him or her through repeated examples and real world incidents.

6. Assisting the supervisee in the development and maintenance of clinical and supervisory records: Record keeping is a vital component of our professional practices, particularly when one realizes the role of adequate record keeping in filing for reimbursement from third party payers. Not only for financial reasons, record keeping is the clinicians' guide to how the client is progressing (or regressing) in the clinical process. Closely aligned with this is the need to assist supervisees in developing skills of verbal and written reports, and editing skills.

7. Interacting with the supervisee in planning, executing, and analyzing supervisory conferences: The supervisory conference is an opportunity for sharing the experiences and perceptions of both the supervisor and the supervisee. Both parties should enter the conference with an open mind to facilitate learning. In addition, both the supervisor and supervisee must have respect for the input of the other. Leith, McNiece, and Fuseiier (1989) developed a Supervisory Clinical Interaction Model (SCIM) that can be used to "illustrate the interactions taking place between the supervisor and the supervisee during clinical teaching" (p. 38).

8. Assisting the supervisee in evaluation of clinical performance: Attention is focused on self-evaluation elsewhere in this chapter. It is very possible that, once a clinician graduates from graduate

school and completes the clinical fellowship year, his or her boss may be of some profession other than speech-language pathology. Therefore, in order to grow and improve as a clinician, the individual needs to have self-evaluation skills.

9. Sharing information regarding ethical, legal, regulatory, and reimbursement aspects of professional practice: With so much information on delays, disorders, and differences one must provide for students in speech-language pathology, it is easy to overlook the legal, moral, and responsibility factors that often govern some of the decision-making that speech-language pathologists must make. Furthermore, speech-language pathologists who are in a supervisory role must, as another supervisory task, model and facilitate professional conduct. This includes exhibiting professional conduct that knows no boundaries amongst professionals, and facilitating professional conduct in supervisees.

10. Demonstrating research skills in the clinical or supervisory process: In recent years ASHA, along with many of the medical professions, has placed a strong emphasis on the use of evidence-based practice, including advocating for the need for increased clinical research. Likewise, supervisor groups in speech-language pathology (including ASHA Special Interest Division: Administration and Supervision) have also emphasized this need for research that validates our supervision methods.

## The Supervisory Conference

In many ways, the interaction between a supervisor and supervisee is very similar to the interaction between client and clinician. The ultimate goal of therapy is for the client to assume responsibility for the use of his or her newly learned information in his or her natural settings. Likewise, supervisors guide supervisees toward independence in applying his or her knowledge in all professional settings.

Dowling lists several factors to consider when planning a supervisory conference. It is critical that the supervisor fully understand the supervisee's needs. In many ways the experience of the supervisee should dictate how much input the supervisor offers versus how much the supervisee brings to the conference. In 1982, Dowling and

Wittkopp conducted a survey of graduate and undergraduate student clinicians at six universities.

> The resulting data identify five valued behaviors in regard to the student conference: (1) regularly scheduled individual conferences; (2) the availability of additional meetings, as needed; (3) active supervisee-supervisor problem-solving in the conference; (4) mutual decisions as to diagnostic and therapeutic techniques; (5) the supervisee's receipt of both positive and negative feedback about their clinical behavior. (Dowling, 2001, p. 121)

The supervisor/supervisee conference that is held immediately following a session with a client should be structured to facilitate the supervisee's self-exploration. "Self-exploration provides opportunities for the clinician to integrate, discover, and develop aspects of his [sic] clinical personality, clinical practice, and technical knowledge" (Oratio, 1977, p. 134). Without this ability to reflect on one's interactions with a client, a supervisee will never be able to become independently capable of assuming "responsibility for clinical judgment and decision making" (Oratio, p. 134). As the supervisee moves along the continuum toward independence, he or she should become involved in planning the conference, and the supervisee should increase the amount of input and self-exploration as the supervisor gradually withdraws from the role of director of the conference.

Conferences do not always have to be individual. At the University of Florida, the supervisors meet with the supervisees weekly as a group where common issues are explored and cases are presented. We also meet individually with our supervisees immediately following their clinical sessions to review the data, discuss the session, review and modify procedures, and facilitate the supervisee's self-analysis of the session, and once again for the student to present his or her therapy plan for the next session and the rationale for his or her clinical decision-making.

We can learn so much from our clients. That is why the first question I have for my supervisees following a session with a client is, "What did you learn from your client today?" Our patients can teach us perseverance. They can teach us patience. They can teach us the importance of "waiting silently." The day we stop learning from our clients is the day that we compromise our being lifelong learners. Continuing education is a daily event; it is not limited to conferences spent listening to experts share their knowledge with us.

## Self-Supervision

Casey, Smith, and Ulrich (1988) define self-supervision as the

> Phase in development where an individual is *independently* capable of planning, observing analyzing, and integrating findings for future application. Functioning independently implies that the individual knows when to seek assistance, where help may be found, how to formulate questions to achieve efficient and effective advice, and further, that the individual is able to accept or reject suggestions appropriately. (p. 23)

Relating self-supervision to the continuum further discussed below:

> *Evaluative/Feedback Stage:* "the active planning to request direction or evaluation, initiating the request, attending to the response, and using the feedback."

> *Transition:* Requesting from the supervisor some "suggestions on how the interaction could be observed and analyzed"

> *Self-Evaluation:* prompts "the supervisee to investigate available information on the topic (e.g., journal articles, texts), select one or two for presentation to the supervisor, actively discuss their pros and cons with the supervisor, and then independently select a methodology for implementation on the basis of the discussion"

Casey, Smith, and Ulrich (1988) listed the following seven purposes for Self-Evaluation:

1. To assess strengths and needs
2. To facilitate development of clinical and supervisory skills
3. To understand clinical interactions (i.e., clinician effect on client behavior and client effect on clinician behavior)
4. To understand intraprofessional (within the profession) interactions (i.e., clinician effects on supervisor and/or colleagues, supervisor effect on clinician or others)
5. To understand interprofessional (outside the profession) interactions (e.g., non-speech-language pathology or audiology supervisor or administrator, or other health care or education professionals)

6. To ensure accountability in both the clinical and supervisory process
7. To understand issues and be aware of resources related to self-supervision.

## Self-Supervision Is on a Continuum of Three Stages

Dowling (n.d.) states that the primary goal of supervision is to develop competent clinicians who are able to self-supervise and self-evaluate. Self-evaluation includes the ability to make accurate clinical diagnoses, and then translate diagnostic results into a viable treatment program; the ability to evaluate clinical management by examining treatment objectives and procedures, the client's behavior, and the clinician's own behavior; the insight to answer the questions "What did I do that facilitated and/or impeded clinical progress?" and the ability to modify his or her own behavior for future sessions. As cited by Casey, Smith, and Ulrich, Anderson (1988) developed a three-stage process to facilitate achieving a level of self-supervision. In the first stage, the evaluation-feedback stage, the supervisor provides direction, feedback, and evaluation, and the supervisee functions primarily as a receiver of the information provided by the supervisor.

The second stage is the transitional stage. In this stage, the supervisee "has acquired sufficient knowledge and skills to be a more active participant in planning, implementing, and evaluating both the clinical and supervisory interaction" (Casey, Smith, & Ulrich, 1988, p. 10). In this transition stage, the supervisor recognizes "the supervisee's emerging competence . . . and facilitates and accepts the supervisee's increasing ability to assume responsibility (Casey, Smith, & Ulrich p. 10).

In the final stage of learning self-supervision, the supervisee assumes the dominant role and is accountable for effectiveness, including responsibility for continued development of clinical skills and professional self-growth (Casey, Smith, & Ulrich, p.10).

The point should be made that it is possible that the supervisee will move back and forth on the continuum. For example, if a client who has aphasia comes in for treatment, the supervisee may need to start at the beginning of the continuum if she has not worked previously with a client with aphasia.

## Utilization and Supervision of Support Personnel

The use of support personnel has emerged as one way to handle the rising costs of health care. However, even though trained paraprofessionals can provide assistance in generalization and maintenance programs, some HMOs/MCOs will not pay unless the services are provided by the highest qualified provider. In addition to the use of support personnel, there has been increased need for family involvement since rehabilitation stays are shorter and outpatient services are curtailed. It is critical for the professional to identify factors in a family that will minimize or maximize follow-through at home.

In 2004, ASHA adopted a position statement on the use of support personnel in speech-language pathology, stressing it supports the use of support personnel, but reminds the speech-language pathologist that "the communication needs and protection of the consumer must be held paramount at all times" (p. 1). ASHA defined support personnel as "people who, following academic and/or on-the-job training, perform tasks as prescribed, directed, and supervised by certified speech-language pathologists" (ASHA, 1995, p. 2; Kayser, 1994, p. 289). The use of support personnel enables a speech-language pathologist to increase the efficiency, availability, and frequency of services provided as long as the personnel are well-trained and well-supervised. However, it should be made clear to a client that when a paraprofessional is providing the services, the speech-language pathologist "retains legal and ethical responsibility for all services provided or omitted" (ASHA, 1995, p. 3). A paraprofessional can conduct speech, language, and/or hearing screenings after having been trained by the supervising clinician. He or she can also provide intervention services that are designed by the supervising clinician, and that do not require any clinical decision-making. Paraprofessionals also can assist in maintaining clinical records, chart recording, and preparation of clinical materials. In no way, however, should a paraprofessional be involved in clinical decision-making, determining eligibility for services, assessing and diagnosing clients, interpreting data, writing assessment or intervention reports, or transmitting clinical information to other professionals (Kayser, 1994).

ASHA recommends that a paraprofessional have an associate's degree, or its equivalent. Aides or paraprofessionals in school settings may have different qualifications and scope of practice depending on the district in which they are hired. A speech-language pathologist should not supervise support personnel until the speech-language pathologist "has completed the ASHA certification examination, the Clinical Fellowship, and two additional years of clinical experience after receiving the Certificate of Clinical Competence in Speech-Language Pathology from ASHA" (ASHA, 1995, p. 42).

With regard to the amount of supervision of paraprofessionals that is deemed necessary and adequate, ASHA recommends that support personnel be supervised for 30% of their first 90 days of employment, with at least 20% of that 30% being direct supervision. Following the first 90 days, supervision should be at a minimum of a 20% level with at least 10% being direct. Direct supervision is defined as "on-site, in-view observation and guidance by a speech-language pathologist while an assigned activity is performed by support personnel" (ASHA, 1995, p. 4). Indirect supervision includes demonstrations, review of audio and/or videotapes, chart reviews, and/or interactive television. They further recommend that each supervisor should supervise no more than three assistants at any one time.

Some school-based clinicians train their paraprofessionals to run computer intervention programs, and to assist in providing classroom-based intervention. However, the supervisor should adhere to the ASHA description or duties for a paraprofessional (Appendix 11B), particularly with regard to scope of practice

Some support personnel fulfill the role of translator or interpreter for clients who have limited English skills. They can assist the clinician in providing therapy in the client's first language if there is a language or speech disorder, or they can serve to facilitate the learning of English as a second language

Suggested competencies for speech-language pathology assistants include interpersonal skills, personal qualities, and technical assistance skills. Skills related to screening and treatment are also suggested. These are summarized in Appendix 11C.

## The Supervisory Process—Providing Feedback

"Feedback is the cornerstone of both growth and productivity." (Anonymous)

## *Purposes of Performance Evaluation*

Golper and Brown (2004) list the purposes of performance evaluation as follows:

- "Express recognition and appreciation for the contributions made by the (supervisee) during the year.
- "Discuss the (supervisee's) performance, including strengths and weaknesses.
- "Address the quality and quantity of the (supervisee's) work.
- "Assess and foster the (supervisee's) potential for further advancement and development.
- "Build and strengthen the supervisor/(supervisee) mentoring relationship.
- "Examine how goals and objectives were met during the previous year.
- "Plan goals and objectives for the coming year" (p. 109).

The goal of this section is to enhance the supervisee's understanding of the importance of being evaluated by supervisors, and to provide supervisor's with guidelines for providing meaningful and useful feedback to their supervisees.

## *Summative Versus Formative Assessment*

Hallowell and Lund (2000) defined a "meaningful assessment" as one that "enhances our education and training missions in specific, practical, measurable ways" and is "oriented toward improving the effectiveness of training and education" (p. 91). Tucker and Stronge (2005) also write about the accountability function which "reflects a commitment to the important professional goals of competence and quality performance. Accountability is typically viewed as summative and relates to judging the effectives of educational services" (pp. 6–7). To that end, there should be ongoing (formative) assessments, and summative (at the conclusion of the experience) assessment as well. Tucker and Stronge (2005) state that "the improvement function generally is considered formative in nature and suggests the need for continuous professional growth and development" (p. 6).

Formative assessments are composed of ongoing evaluation of performance. They should focus on identifying what goals have been mastered and developing goals to be accomplished prior to the next time of formative assessments. Formative assessments are best implemented in a format that facilitates the learning of self-evaluation, possibly including the supervisees' developing a portfolio that contains the results of formative evaluations, and comparisons of the results of self-evaluation compared to the supervisee's evaluation from his or her supervisors. The portfolio should also include the supervisee's resume, sample projects and/or papers done on the job, and a self-reflective section summarizing the supervisee's accomplishments but, more importantly, reflecting goals the supervisee has developed for his or her own professional growth (Richardson, 2000).

Summative assessments are a final measure of a supervisee's skills and knowledge. In speech-language pathology, ongoing evaluations of a supervisee's progress would constitute formative assessments. The Praxis exam is an example of a summative assessment. Summative assessment typically is done at the completion of a specific activity, with some of the focus being on identifying learning goals for subsequent placements.

### Comparing Evaluative and Objective Feedback

Feedback is provided by one's supervisor or boss as a manner of assessing a supervisee's performance on the job and formulating goals for the supervisee. Evaluative feedback is the most traditional manner of feedback, and is frequently warranted in the early stages of a supervisee's employment. However, in providing evaluative feedback, the supervisor is in a position of judging the appropriateness of the clinician's behavior and performance. Evaluative feedback is appropriate in the early stages of the supervisee's employment, but should not be overused. When an employer assumes a judging posture, self-evaluation by the clinician is discouraged. An example of evaluative feedback is, "You did not engage the child in the activities you designed."

The advantages of evaluative feedback are numerous. Supervisees report that they are motivated more by evaluative feedback than objective feedback, and that evaluative feedback reinforces learning better than objective feedback. It also reinforces mastery of basic information, and "provides clear statements about strengths and weaknesses." This type of feedback also encourages self-competition (Farmer & Farmer, 1959 as cited in Schwab 2002).

On the other hand, supervisors can offer objective feedback. Objective feedback is not valuative, and is not judgmental. Rather, it is based on facts that can be measured as in, "You elicited 15 spontaneous utterances from the child" or "You said 'OK' 22 times during the session." Objective feedback should be the goal for the supervisor as the supervisee progresses. The use of objective feedback is more likely to facilitate reflection by having the supervisee re-evaluate and learn from his or her experiences. Objective feedback can be positive or negative, but supervisors are encouraged to consider the impact of negative feedback on the student's self-confidence, self-esteem, and anxiety levels. (McAllister & Lincoln, 2004). Pfeiffer and Jones (1972) emphasize the importance of objective data rather than evaluative statements because evaluative statements frequently include a "should," which makes the student more defensive.

It is always good to give written feedback because it can serve as a record of the employee's growth (or lack thereof) on the job. Written feedback should include observation data, and a little bit of direct evaluation. It should always be followed up with a discussion between the supervisor and supervisee to explain the purpose and content of the feedback. The written evaluation's message is critical in facilitating a collaborative approach. By giving the supervisee written feedback immediately following a session, the supervisee's analysis prior to the oral conference is enhanced. Written objective feedback should enhance self-analysis and self-evaluation; if the feedback is evaluative, the opportunity to motivate the supervisee to participate in such activities may be lost (McCrea & Brasseur, 2003). When writing feedback, it is suggested that the supervisor write a list of questions, not statements, because questions will facilitate reflection on the session by the supervisee (Dowling, 2001). Runyan and Seal (1985) and Peaper and Mercaitis (1987) analyzed written feedback and found that 40 to 46% of the statements written by the supervisor were evaluative. McCrea and Brasseur (2003) posit that evaluative feedback does not encourage self-analysis and creative thinking; both skills are essential in the development of professionalism.

The amount and type of feedback should follow a continuum, with the supervisee receiving less feedback as he or she gains more experience. In addition, as the supervisee progresses, feedback should be based on objective statements instead of evaluative feedback (Anderson, 1988).

Farmer and Farmer (1988), as cited by Schwab (2002), list four advantages of evaluative feedback:

- It motivates supervisees more than does objective feedback.
- It reinforces learning more than objective feedback does.
- It reinforces mastery of basic information.
- It provides lucid statements about the supervisee's strengths and weaknesses.

In contrast, Schwab (2002) lists four advantages of objective feedback.

- It is based on the supervisor's observations.
- It is not judgmental, so the supervisee is more likely to follow up on suggestions made by the supervisor.
- It is verifiable because it is based on factual data.
- It enhances the ability of the supervisee to self-evaluate by analyzing the data collected and problem-solve. The ultimate goal in this process is for the supervisee to make his or her own decisions.

In summary, there are strengths and weaknesses of both objective and evaluative feedback. It is up to the supervisor to monitor the types of feedback he or she provides to the supervisee and its effects on subsequent clinician/client interactions, and to guide the supervisee along the continuum to the point of being able to self-evaluate and set goals based on that evaluation.

### Guidelines for Giving Feedback

The primary job of a supervisor is not to just observe the supervisee, but to offer constructive feedback to the supervisee. Feedback can be objective and facilitate the supervisee's eventual ability to self-evaluate. It can consist of evaluative comments, comments based on objective data gathered during the observation, suggestions, and questions. First and most importantly, it is absolutely critical for the supervisor to offer a balance of positive and negative feedback. This will allow for emotional support as well as a foundation for future goals and performance guidelines following the feedback.

A second rule is to avoid emotional language. Emotional language can put the supervisee into a defensive mode and may lead to challenges by the supervisee as to the accuracy of the supervisor's perceptions in light of a lack of objective data. This leads to a third guideline, that is, to use data collection to support your observations as supervisor.

Fourth, the feedback offered to the supervisee should focus on the impact of the clinicians' behaviors on the client. For example, the supervisor observed a therapy session conducted by a speech-language pathologist who was doing her clinical fellowship year in which the clinician had gone into a 50-minute session with a four-year-old with nothing but a deck of cards depicting target sounds and the concepts of over/under. The clinician showed very little affect other than frustration when the child refused to stay in his seat, eventually sliding out of his chair (that was backed up into a corner) and taking up residence under the table (and the clinician failed to take advantage of the opportunity to reinforce the concept of "under" that the client had provided!). In the follow-up conference in which the supervisor provided primarily evaluative feedback, the clinician became defensive and did not take responsibility for the misguided session.

A fifth guideline is for the supervisor to be specific and give examples of behaviors that have been observed. When the supervisor in the previous scenario turned away from evaluative statements and began to objectively analyze the session, the supervisee was a bit more receptive and responsive without getting more defensive. The supervisor and supervisee then followed a sixth rule, which is to suggest possible options, and to pose questions that will lead the supervisee into analyzing the session's strengths and weaknesses and enhance self-evaluation.

### Criteria for Effective Feedback

Swan (1991) writes that, regardless of whether one is offering objective or evaluative feedback, the supervisor should strive to create a stage for future discussions. To that end, one of Swan's suggestions is to say, "From my perspective . . ." instead of "I'll show you where you were wrong." (p. 159). In her book, *Supervision: Strategies for Successful Outcomes and Productivity*, Dowling (2001) cites Pfeiffer and

Jones' (1972) listing of characteristics of effective feedback. These characteristics are as follows:

- Descriptive
- Specific (The greater the specificity, the more helpful the feedback.)
- Responsive to needs of the system
- Oriented to modifiable behavior
- Solicited rather than imposed
- Well-timed
- Validated with supervisee

Recall that Pfeiffer and Jones emphasize the importance of objective data rather than evaluative statements because evaluative statements tend to make the supervisee more defensive. In addition, nonspecific (global) information frequently is not meaningful to the supervisee, leaving the supervisee unclear as to what the supervisor was trying to convey. Dowling (1992) makes a crucial statement in writing, "Feedback in areas beyond the individual's current ability to modify was without value" (p. 115).

With regard to not imposing feedback on the supervisee, the supervisor should establish a relationship with the supervisee that leads to a "comfort zone" in which the supervisee can request feedback. Requested feedback is always more productive than imposed feedback.

The timing of delivering feedback is also crucial. Immediate feedback (as opposed to delayed) typically is more efficient as the session being evaluated just occurred and is fresh in the minds of both supervisor and supervisee. As a supervisor in a university clinic, I make written notes of my observations and sit down with the supervisee immediately after the session to review the session. I pose questions that can provide the supervisee an opportunity to reflect on the session, analyze it, and make proposals for changes in future sessions.

Freeman (1985) makes a similar listing of considerations in providing effective feedback: systematicity, timeliness (reasonable turnaround time between the end of the observation and the provision of feedback to the supervisee), understandability, acceptability, and reciprocity. Systematicity involves having the supervisor react to what he or she observes. "Inconsistency from observation to observation may occur in terms of volume and the aspects of behavior singled out for comment. To deal with this issue, professional objectives for the supervisee, requests for specific types of feedback from the supervisee, and preselection of a specific goal for observation will help structure the narrative" (p.78). Understandability and reciprocity are closely associated when writing a narrative report. The supervisor "needs to take care that the content conveys what is intended. The information and observations must be sufficiently complete and coherent to be accurately interpreted by the supervisee" (p. 79).

## Involving the Supervisee

Crago (1987) suggests having the supervisee evaluate the supervisor's feedback in terms of how helpful the comments were. This will enable the supervisee to reflect on the supervisor's feedback and to let him or her know the value of specific comments, thereby cuing the supervisor as to what types of comments that particular supervisee most benefits from. The supervisor can then adjust his or her style to fit more closely with the supervisee's learning style.

In guiding the supervisee to the process of self-evaluation, Crago (1987) suggests having the supervisee write down one successful aspect of the session, one unsuccessful aspect, and one "surprise" aspect. The supervisor can take the list generated by the supervisee and use it as a "jumping off point" for the supervisory conference following a clinic session with a client. Along the same lines, Dowling (2001) suggests listing events that are representative of the supervisee's strengths, and reflective of weaknesses for each observation.

Another way to actively involve the supervisee in the supervision process is to write a list of questions upon which the supervisee can reflect instead of making a list of statements. Also, in an effort not to overwhelm the supervisee too much, avoid addressing too many issues at one time. Initially, address two to three problems that have the most effect on the client's behaviors; when they are understood and implemented, identify the next set of problems/goals to address with the supervisee. With regard to "acceptability," the supervisor should take care not to overwhelm the supervisee with feedback while maintaining a balance between positive and negative feedback, thus facilitating the supervisee's acceptance of the feedback.

## Comparing Oral and Written Feedback

In 1987, Peaper and Mercaitis asked the following three questions to compare verbal interactions and written feedback:

1. What is the nature of narrative feedback written by supervisors while observing a session?
2. How do the patterns of written feedback compare with patterns of verbal interaction described in previous studies of a previous conference?
3. Does the nature of written feedback vary with increased supervisory experience?

As reported by Peaper and Mercaitis (1987), in 1977 Culatta and Selzer "studied 12 weeks of supervisory conferences and found that only 9% of the responses were evaluative in nature with two thirds of the evaluation statements being made by the supervisor." Peaper and Mercaitis (1987) also cite Roberts and Smith (1982) who determined that oral conferences are more analytical than they are evaluative.

Peaper and Mercaitis (1987) identified six types of statements in written feedback:

- Good evaluation (supervisor approved of the observed behavior)
- Bad evaluation (supervisor gave disapproval of the observed behavior)
- Question (any interrogative statement made by the supervisor relevant to the session)
- Strategy (any statement by the supervisor to the supervisee with regard to future therapeutic intervention)
- Observation/information (any relevant comment that is not evaluating, questioning, or providing strategy)
- Irrelevant (any statement with no direct relationship to the therapy session)

They also found that evaluative comments in written feedback constituted 40% of the comments as opposed to 9% in the oral conferences. This correlates with the findings of Runyan and Seal (1985) who found that 46% of the comments written by supervisors as they observed a session were evaluative. In 1987, Peaper and Mercaitis found essentially the same thing with 40% of the comments being evaluative in nature. McCrea and Brasseur (2003) addressed two implications based on these findings.

> This propensity toward evaluation suggests that many supervisors perceive evaluation as their primary role. Although this supervisor-as-evaluator role is consistent with the Direct-Active style, it is incongruent with the Collaborative and Consultative styles. (p. 160)

> Regardless of intent, supervisors' written comments tend to be highly evaluative (Peaper & Mercaitis, 1987; Runyan & Seal, 1985). As stated previously, it is these active, direct behaviors of the supervisor that do not encourage, in fact probably discourage, self-analysis and creative thinking on part of supervisees. (p. 167)

The author of this book collected samples of written feedback from approximately 40 supervisors in university clinics. Each statement on the feedback was coded as one of the six types identified by Peaper and Mercaitis. The results are outlined in Table 11–3.

Peaper and Mercaitis (1987) provide a percentage breakdown of comments based on the number of years of supervisor experience. These findings are delineated in Table 11–4.

### What Does the Business World Have to Say About Feedback?

In reviewing the medical and business literature, the author found different perspectives on feedback. In the business literature, Hawley (2004) said that effective narratives should include the following:

- Helping the employee identify barriers to success
- Defining a timeline during which one can expect correction of the performance
- Providing "coaching, counseling, support, and tools from management to aid in successful rehabilitation" (p. 37).
- Keeping two-way communication open after the initial written feedback
- Providing positive reinforcement along the way to improvement

**Table 11-3.** Examples of Types of Evaluative Feedback

| Type of Written Feedback | % Statements | Example |
|---|---|---|
| Good evaluation | 30.6% | Good to use the tongue depressor to provide tactile input. It helped! |
| Bad evaluation | 9.4% | You played the game too long at the expense of getting only a few spontaneous utterances. |
| Question | 9.6% | Is it prosody, tongue carriage, rate, or something else that is interfering with his intelligibility? |
| Strategy | 26.0% | Don't forget to use a mirror and the SeeScape. I think this would help him. |
| Observation/ Information | 24.3% | He's saying the name of the letter /r/ on "red." Maybe spend some time talking about the difference between a letter's name and its sound." |
| Irrelevant | 0.1% | Remind me to get that book out of Dr. Smith's office. |

**Table 11-4.** Breakdown of Feedback Statements Based on Supervisor's Years of Experience

| Yrs. of Experience | Good Evaluation | Bad Evaluation | Question | Strategy | Obs/ Info |
|---|---|---|---|---|---|
| 0–2 | **42.1%** | 11% | 2.7% | 21.7% | 22.4% |
| 2+ –4 | **29.1%** | 10.9% | 8.8% | 25.1% | 25.8% |
| 4+ –6 | 22.3% | 6.2% | **28.1%** | 25.1% | 18.5% |
| +6 | 26.2% | 8.5% | 9.8% | **29.3%** | 26% |

Hawley (2004) developed a "Feedback Skills Checklist" to guide supervisors in providing feedback:

- Focus on the positive first
- Focus on behaviors, not personalities
- Be hard on the problem but gentle on the person
- Be descriptive and constructive, not judgmental and evaluative
- Use positive or neutral language
- If you have to be critical, explain where improvements can be made in the future.

Weiss (1988) also compared written and oral feedback. Weiss maintains that written communications have a major weakness compared to oral feedback in that the supervisee cannot ask questions, or there is a delay between receiving the narrative feedback and meeting with the supervisor to review the narrative. Weiss also suggests that the supervisor carefully review his or her written feedback prior to giving it to the supervisee, "read(ing) it back as if you were the reader to make certain that it conveys the request or information you intended" (p. 120).

## What Do Medical Educators Have to Say About Feedback?

Elnicki, Layne, Ogden, and Morris (1998) studied the effects of written versus oral feedback on clinical performance of 68 internal medicine residents. They found that there were no differences on the students' performance as differentiated by the oral versus written feedback groups. Elnicki et al. stated that medical educators should focus more on the level of detail and frequency of feedback than on the form of the feedback. They also broke down the percentage of comments based on supervisory experience as shown in Table 11–5. Supervisors with the least amount of experience tended to be evaluative, whereas it took over 4 years for supervisors or students in the medical setting to use the more productive techniques of questions and strategies. The author hopes that by presenting this information to supervisors in speech-language pathology, they will implement the better feedback strategies from the beginning of their supervisory experiences.

**Table 11–5.** Number of Years of Supervisory Experience and Percentage of Good Evaluation Statements

| No. Yrs. Supervisory Experience | % of Comments |
|---|---|
| 0–2 years | 42.1% of comments were good evaluation statements |
| 2+ –4 years | 29.1% of comments were good evaluation statements |
| 4+ –6 years | 28.1% were questions |
| 6+ years | 29.3% were strategies |

*Source:* Elnicki, Layve, Ogden, & Norris (1998).

Markus, Mast, and Soler (1980) studied the effects of different types of feedback on examinations of medical students by comparing performance on later cumulative exams on the same information. Their results showed that statistically, there was little difference on retest performance between the students who received written feedback and the students who received oral feedback on the original examinations. However, when they asked the students what type of feedback they preferred, 59% of the students preferred written feedback, 16% preferred oral feedback, and 24% found both modes to be useful. In conclusion to their study, Markus et al. said the following:

> Faculty must weigh other values in selecting between oral and written feedback. An hour spent writing elaborated feedback is appreciated by students and provides them with a useful study guide for future references; an hour spent in an oral review session offers an opportunity for insight into a student's reasoning processes and for listening to students' concerns. The oral review session also gives the instructor insight into the quality of his test questions by creating an open forum atmosphere in which students can argue the subtle points of each question and can identify ambiguities in items that were not noticed before. (p. 791)

## The Objective Narrative

Swan (1991) advocates for writing an appraisal of one's supervisees using what he calls "the objective narrative." Swan enumerates a three-step process for writing an appraisal based on the collection of three types of data. The first is objective data; the second is significant incidences (positive and negative; can include observations such as showing initiative, problem-solving using an analytical approach); the third are the behaviors the supervisor observes when managing the supervisee. When the observed session(s) have taken place, the supervisor should (1) gather and analyze the data throughout the appraisal period, (2) rate the performance, and (3) write the narrative portions of the appraisal. Whether written or oral, Swan maintains that each objective should be rated, that each performance factor should be rated, and an overall summary rating should be provided. As have many others writing on performance evaluations, Swan maintains that it is not about rewards and punishments. The goal should be to facilitate problem-solving any problems that have been identified in the appraisal process. Instead of saying, "I'll show you where you are wrong," Swan writes that the supervisor should say, "From my perspective . . . " This change in phrasing helps to set a tone of "reasonableness" and sets the stage for subsequent discussions.

In writing objective narratives, it is critical that the supervisor use written documentation throughout the appraisal period to help answer two questions:

- "What is my evidence for performance on each objective?
- "Why is it done that way?" (as opposed to "What do I remember, what do I think of, how do I think they did, do I like them or not?)

Before writing an objective narrative, the supervisor should have gathered numerous (8–12) objective pieces of data plus a critical incidence or two. With this much data on hand, the supervisor can say with confidence, " 'Obviously, the evidence supports the conclusion that this person overall is meeting the standard I set' or 'I can see plenty of evidence that they're way above or way below the standard.' Whatever my conclusion may be, the evidence is there" (Swan, p. 130).

## Summary

Rosenzweig, Kast, and Mitchell (1991) describe the main goal in appraising a supervisee's performance as being "to compare actual results with desired results and to design action plans that will close any gaps" (p. 70). To criticize a supervisee is counter productive unless the criticism is concurrent with action planning and goal setting. Ideally, the supervisee would initiate the action planning and goal setting. If not, the supervisor can propose the actions and goals, and assist the supervisee in accepting them. "The test of a feedback system is not whether or not it measures successfully, but whether or not it induces changes in behavior" of the supervisee (Maister, 1993, p. 84). McAllister and Lincoln (2004) write that "a well-conducted assessment should leave students (supervisees) feeling happy and proud of their achievements, aware of their weaknesses, and focused on specific areas of practice to address in the next placement" (p. 149).

The development of the goals to be accomplished over a period of time needs to be a joint responsibility of the clinician and the supervisor. Likewise, the achievement of those end goals is a shared responsibility between the supervisee and the supervisor. Ultimately, end goals should be designed to facilitate the development of professional self-supervision, and to guide self-growth through the supervisory process. Of course, one would assume that the development of clinical skills that are designed to ensure the delivery of quality clinical services is utmost in the eyes of the supervisor and supervisee (Casey, Smith, & Ulrich, 1988).

## References

American Speech-Language-Hearing Association. (1985). Clinical supervision in speech-language pathology and audiology: A position statement. *Asha*, 27(6), 57–60.

American Speech-Language-Hearing Association (1995, December). Guidelines for the training and credentialing, use, and supervision of speech-language pathology assistants. *Asha*, 37, 1–10.

American Speech-Language-Hearing Association. (2004). *Training, use, and Supervision of support personnel in speech-language pathology* [Position statement]. Available from www.asha.org/policy

Anderson, J. L. (1988). *The supervisory process in speech-language pathology and audiology.* Boston: Little, Brown.

Casey, P. L., Smith, K. J., & Ulrich, S. R. (1988). *Self-supervision: A career tool for audiologists and speech-language pathologists.* NSSLHA's Clinical Series No. 10. Rockville, MD: American Speech-Language-Hearing Association.

Cogan, M. (1973). *Clinical supervision.* Boston: Houghton-Mifflin.

Crago, M. (1987). Supervision and self-exploration. In M. Crago & M. Pickering (Eds.), *Supervision in human communication disorders: Perspectives on a process* (pp. 137-167). San Diego, CA: Singular.

Culatta, R., & Selzer, H. (1977). Content and sequence analysis of the supervisory session: A report of clinical use. *Asha, 19,* 523-526.

Dowling, S. (1992). *Implementing the supervisory process: Theory and practice.* Englewood Cliffs, NJ: Prentice-Hall.

Dowling, S. (2001). *Supervision: Strategies for successful outcomes and productivity.* Needham Heights, MA: Allyn & Bacon.

Elnicki, D. M., Layne, R. D., Ogden, P. E., & Morris, D. K. (1998). Oral versus written feedback in medical clinic. *Journal of General Internal Medicine, 13*(3), 155-158.

Farmer, S., & Farmer, J. (1989). *Supervision in communication disorders.* Columbus, OH: Merrill.

Freeman, E. (1985). The importance of feedback in clinical supervision: Implications for direct practice. *Clinical Supervisor, 3*(1), 5-26.

Glatthorn, A. (1984). *A differentiated supervision.* Alexandria, VA: Association for Supervision and Curriculum Development.

Golper, L. A. C., & Brown, J. E. (2004). *Business matters: A guide for speech-language pathologists.* Rockville Pike, MD: American Speech-Language-Hearing Association.

Hallowell, B. (2000). Formative and summative assessments: Doing it with meaning. In *Council of Academic Programs in Communication Sciences and Disorders proceedings of the annual conference* (pp. 91-99). Minneapolis, MN: Council of Academic Programs in Communication Sciences and Disorders.

Hallowell, B., & Lund, N. (1998). Fostering program improvements through a focus on educational outcomes proceedings: In P. S. Murphy, R. McGuire, & L. Bliss (Eds.), *Proceedings of the Annual Conference on Graduate Education* (pp. 32-61). Minneapolis, MN: Council of Academic Programs in Communication Sciences and Disorders.

Hawley, C. F. (2004). *201 ways to turn any employee into a star performer.* Columbus, OH: McGraw Hill.

Kayser, H. (1994). Service delivery issues for multicultural populations. In R. Lubinski & C. Frattali, *Professional issues in speech-language pathology and audiology* (pp. 282-292). San Diego, CA: Singular.

Leith, W. R., McNiece, E. M., & Fusilier, B. B. (1989). *Handbook of supervision: A cognitive behavioral system.* Boston: Little, Brown.

Maister, D. H. (1993). *Managing the professional service firm.* New York: Free Press Paperbacks.

McAllister, L., & Lincoln, M. (2004). *Clinical education in speech-language pathology.* Philadelphia: Whurr.

Markus, J. F., Mast, T. A., & Soler, N. G. (1980). The effects of written and oral feedback following examinations. *Journal of Medical Education, 55*(9), 790-792.

McCrea, E. S., & Brasseur, J. A. (2003). *The supervisory process in speech-language pathology and audiology.* Boston: Allyn & Bacon.

Oratio, A. R. (1977). *Supervision in speech pathology: A handbook for supervisors and clinicians.* Baltimore: University Park Press.

Peaper, R., & Mercaitis, P. (1987). The nature of narrative written feedback provided to student clinicians: A descriptive study. In S. Farmer (Ed.), *Proceedings of a national conference on supervision-clinical supervision: A coming of age.* Council of University Supervisors of Practicum in Speech-Language Pathology and Audiology, Jekyll Island, GA.

Pfeiffer, J., & Jones, J. (1972). Openness: Collusion and feedback. *The 1972 annual handbook of group facilitators* (pp. 197-201). Tucson, AZ: University Associates.

Richardson, K. (2000). Formative and summative assessments in an Au.D. program. In *Council of Academic Programs in Communication Sciences and Disorders Proceedings of the Annual Conference* (pp. 116-128). Minneapolis, MN: Council of Academic Programs in Communication Sciences and Disorders.

Rosenzweig, J., Kast, F., & Mitchell, T. R. (1991). *The frank and earnest manager.* Los Altos, CA: Crisp.

Runyan, S., & Seal, B. (1985). A comparison of supervisors' ratings while observing a language remediation session. *The Clinical Supervisor, 3,* 61-75.

Schwab, W. S. (2002, May). *Personality, supervisory process and written feedback in the clinical setting.* Greensboro, NC. Unpublished paper.

Swan, W. S. (1991). *How to do a superior performance appraisal.* New York: John Wiley & Sons.

Tucker, P. D., & Stronge, J. H. (2005). *Linking teacher evaluation and student learning.* Alexandria: Virginia Association for Supervision and Curriculum Development.

Weiss, W. H. (1988). *Supervisor's standard reference handbook* (2nd ed.). Englewood Cliffs, NJ: Prentice-Hall.

## APPENDIX 11A
## Supervisor's and Supervisee's Bill of Rights*

A group of 31 speech pathologists and 8 individuals from other professions met in March, 1976 to define a "Bill of Rights" for supervisors and supervisees. The result of this meeting was to define reasonable expectations for both supervisors and supervisees in the workplace. Although it was not designed to cover the supervision of students in university settings, some of the items can be applied to that setting as well.

## Supervisee's Bill of Rights

I. Right to an Adequate Physical Working Environment (Not Always Under Supervisor's Control)

II. Right to Expect Certain Characteristics of Supervisor
   A. To have educational qualifications—meet CCC standards with well rounded or appropriate clinical experience
   B. To be flexible in allowing the supervisee to explore different methods of therapy than he currently possesses.
   C. To be dynamic and motivating
   D. To be confident (not defensive), fair, and flexible.
   E. To be consistent in values.
   F. To be sensitive to individual as a whole, realizing both personal and professional needs and differences.
   G. To guide but encourage independence.
   H. To provide atmosphere for creativity, learning, and research
   I. To know limitations.
   J. To differentiate between personal preferences and objective criticism.
   K. To be dependable.
   L. To demonstrate availability and organization.
   M. To encourage and stimulate professional growth.
      1. To assist the supervisee to make job more creative—"Job ladder" is limited in field.
      2. To provide options of which supervisee is unaware.

*Reprinted with permission from: Supervisory relationships: Experiences in dynamic communication, *Asha*, *19*(8), 527–529. Copyright 1977 by American Speech-Language-Hearing Association. All rights reserved.

3. To expand responsibilities with growing expertise and personal goals.
4. To provide realistic opportunities for research, expand expertise in another area.

N. To expect supervisor to be responsible for organization and management concerns affecting the supervisee and act as coordinator among the director, staff, students, and Clinical Fellowship Year (CFY) candidates.

III. Right to Expect Supervisor to Provide Means and Method of Feedback with:
   A. Systematic monitoring
   B. Ongoing mutual feedback.
   C. Opportunity to express self (opinions, recommendations).
   D. Formal and informal conference time.
   E. Hones appraisal of job performance.
   F. Oral and written evaluations.
   G. Possibility of appealing decisions.
   H. Opportunity to say "No."

IV. Right to Specific Role Definition
   A. To accept responsibility in the job description to include:
      1. Awareness of clinical policies and regulations.
      2. Clear-cut definitions.
         a, To help establish written criteria for supervision.
         b. To negotiate "rules."
   B. To expect supervisor to communicate expectations from the onset of CFY, on both the long-term and short-term levels.
   C. To question requirements of supervisor.
   D. To disagree with supervisor.
   E. To expect expansion and consideration of special interests when at particular facility for long time.
   F. To further own professional goals within framework of position and responsibilities.
   G. To maintain own individuality while fulfilling job responsibilities.
   H. To select cases in terms of own strengths and preferences when practical.
   I. To receive input regarding caseload selection and time use, for example, caseload, staffings, report writing, conferences.

    J.  To achieve autonomy of expression with appropriate rationale.
    K.  To receive justifiable explanations for supervisor's actions regarding running of clinic or center.
    L.  To expect leadership from supervisor.
        1.  To provide time allocations.
        2.  To specific types of supervision (direct/indirect).
        3.  To provide general procedures, orientation, job description, goals, philosophy.
        4.  To provide professional support.
        5.  To provide support and reinforcement at all levels.
        6.  To provide appropriate observation time.
    M.  To be treated as a professional in training and to be accorded responsibilities congruent with level of training.
    N.  To expect supervisor to be open and tolerant of errors.
    O.  To make mistakes.
    P.  To inform supervisor of difficulties.
    Q.  To expect individual treatment in dealing with work-related problems.
    R.  To refuse certain client management dues to decreased effectiveness in providing service.

  V.  Right to Definition of Grievance Procedure
    A.  To know hierarchy of supervisors.
    B.  To define right to appeal complaints.

## Supervisors' Bill of Rights

  I.  Right to Define General Goals of Center
    A.  To determine quality of work the person feels represents goals of institution.
    B.  To become aware of expectations from the onset of the CFY or employment and to assume the responsibility to communicate this to the supervisee.
    C.  To expect services specifically related to needs of center and relate these to supervisee from beginning.
    D.  To consider expertise and goals of staff.
    E.  To continually re-evaluate needs of center.
    F.  To periodically reevaluate expectations and performance.

G. To redefine services when needs of center change.

II. Right to Describe and Expect Fulfillment of Supervisee's Job Responsibilities
   A. 1. To accept responsibility for arranging and discussing job description.
      2. To be aware and to clearly define clinical policies and regulations.
      3. To know what cases supervisee is expected to work with and how the cases are generally to be managed.
      4. To give supervisee choice of whether the clinician wants more experience with cases not generally seen (offer extra assistance in such cases.)
      5. To know types of exposure clinician has had in other facilities and gaps in experience.
   B. To determine size and type of caseload.
   C. To expect staff's acceptance of exposure to various cases (especially if student).
   D. To tell supervisee not to work with a case any more.
   E. To make final decisions for case management (split after CFY when clinician assumes greater responsibility).
   F. To assume final rights for decision making in work environment, that is, authority of position.
   G. Not to make a decision
   H. 1. To evaluate each patient and client.
      2. To determine procedure/program for each therapy session—written or unwritten short-range goals and long-range goals.
      3. To report on each therapy session.
      4. To assume increasing responsibility from students, CFY interns, and staff:
         a. To participate in decision making in cases.
         b. To have complete responsibility of case history, evaluations, and reports.
         c. To arrange appropriate referrals—that is, to professionals in education, physicians, and psychologists.
      5. To do systematic monitoring.
      6. To know supervisee's goals.
      7. To make alternative suggestions, demands.

8. To question why clinicians are doing what they are doing.
9. To toss duties back to supervisee.

III. Right to be Respected as a Human Being and a Professional
   A. To be honest.
   B. To react emotionally.
   C. To criticize as well as praise.
   D. To expect professional honesty and dependability.
   E. 1. To expect staff to show initiative and questioning of ideas.
      2. To define your rights.
   F. To have legal protection.
   G. To provide model (for students particularly) for clinical and professional actions.
   H. To be receptive and responsive in pursuing various aspects of professional growth.
   I. To expect supervisee to perform in a certain manner, level of behavior, and performance.
      1. To behave professionally.
      2. To be open to constructive criticism, suggestions, guidance.
      3. To determine flexibility.
      4. To use time constructively and applicably.
      5. To distinguish the difference in personal and professional responsibilities.
      6. To know limitations.

IV. Right to Offer and Get Mutual Feedback
   A. To make justified criticism.
   B. To expect staff to expect and accept criticism.
   C. To judge and criticize effect of services, honestly criticize and suggest other ways of operating.
   D. To get feedback from supervisee about supervision received.
   E. To expect supervisee to say, "You're a lousy supervisor," or even a good one.
   F. To determine some of ground rules of how often observed.

V. Right to Establish Mode of Interaction
   A. To create atmosphere of open communication concerning job as well as interpersonal relationships that affect job.

    B.  To create atmosphere for discussion and disagreement.

    C.  To create atmosphere for initiative, motivation, and creativity.

    D.  To avoid "hidden agendas"—be direct!

    E.  To create atmosphere for flexibility.

    F.  To create atmosphere for encouraging supervisee to seek assistance and guidance when needed.

    G.  To be sensitive to individual needs and bring up individual problems.

    H.  To expect that personal problems should not affect work performance.

## APPENDIX 11B
## Competencies for Effective Clinical Supervision*

1.0 **Task:** Establishing and maintaining an effective working relationship with the supervisee

**Competencies required:**

1.1 Ability to facilitate an understanding of the clinical and supervisory processes.

1.2 Ability to organize and provide information regarding the logical sequences of supervisory interaction, that is, joint setting of goals and objectives, data collection and analysis, evaluation.

1.3 Ability to interact from a contemporary perspective with the supervisee in both the clinical and supervisory processes.

1.4 Ability to apply learning principles in the supervisory process.

1.5 Ability to apply skills of interpersonal communication in the supervisory process.

1.6 Ability to facilitate independent thinking and problem-solving by the supervisee.

1.7 Ability to maintain a professional and supportive relationship that allows supervisor and supervisee growth.

1.8 Ability to interact with the supervisee objectively.

1.9 Ability to establish joint communications regarding expectations and responsibilities in the clinical and supervisory processes.

1.10 Ability to evaluate, with the supervisee, the effectiveness of the ongoing supervisory relationship.

2.0 **Task:** Assisting the supervisee in developing clinical goals and objectives.

---

*Reprinted with permission from American Speech-Language-Hearing Association. Committee on Speech-Language Pathology and Audiology. "Clinical supervision in speech-language pathology and audiology: A position statement." *Asha, 27,* 57–60. Copyright 1985 American Speech-Language-Hearing Association. All rights reserved.

**Competencies required:**

2.1  Ability to assist the supervisee in planning effective client goals and objectives.

2.2  Ability to plan, with the supervisee, effective goals and objectives for clinical and professional growth.

2.3  Ability to assist the supervisee in using observation and assessment in preparation of client goals and objectives.

2.4  Ability to assist the supervisee in using self-analysis and previous evaluation in preparation of goals and objectives for professional growth.

2.5  Ability to assist the supervisee in assigning priorities to clinical goals and objectives.

2.6  Ability to assist the supervisee in assigning priorities to goals and objectives for professional growth.

3.0  **Task:** Assisting the supervisee in developing and refining assessment skills.

**Competencies required:**

3.1  Ability to share current research findings and evaluation procedures in communication disorders.

3.2  Ability to facilitate an integration of research findings and evaluation procedures in communication disorders.

3.3  Ability to assist the supervisee in providing rationale for assessment procedures.

3.4  Ability to assist supervisee in communicating assessment procedures and rationales.

3.5  Ability to assist the supervisee in integrating findings and observations to make appropriate recommendations.

4.0  **Task:** Assisting the supervisee in developing and refining management skills.

**Competencies required:**

4.1  Ability to share current research findings and management procedures in communication disorders.

4.2　Ability to facilitate an integration of research findings in client management.

4.3　Ability to assist the supervisee in providing rationale for treatment procedures.

4.4　Ability to assist the supervisee in identifying appropriate sequences for client change.

4.5　Ability to assist the supervisee in adjusting steps in the progression toward a goal.

4.6　Ability to assist the supervisee in the description and measurement of client and clinician change.

4.7　Ability to assist the supervisee in documenting client and clinician change.

4.8　Ability to assist the supervisee in integrating documented client and clinician change to evaluate progress and specify future recommendations.

5.0　**Task:** Demonstrating for and participating with the supervisee in the clinical process.

**Competencies required:**

5.1　Ability to determine jointly when demonstration is appropriate.

5.2　Ability to demonstrate or participate in an effective client-clinician relationship.

5.3　Ability to demonstrate a variety of clinical techniques and participate with the supervisee in clinical management.

5.4　Ability to demonstrate or use jointly the specific materials and equipment of the profession.

5.5　Ability to demonstrate or participate jointly in counseling of clients or family/guardians of clients.

6.0　**Task:** Assisting the supervisee in observing and analyzing assessment and treatment sessions.

**Competencies required:**

6.1　Ability to assist the supervisee in learning a variety of data collection procedures.

6.2　Ability to assist the supervisee in selecting and executing data collection procedures.

6.3 Ability to assist the supervisee in accurately recording data.

6.4 Ability to assist the supervisee in analyzing and interpreting data objectively.

6.5 Ability to assist the supervisee in revising plans for client management based on data obtained.

7.0 **Task:** Assisting the supervisee in development and maintenance of clinical and supervisory records.

**Competencies required:**

7.1 Ability to assist the supervisee in applying record-keeping systems in supervisory and clinical processes.

7.2 Ability to assist the supervisee in effectively document-ing supervisory and clinically related interactions.

7.3 Ability to assist the supervisee in organizing records to facilitate easy retrieval of information concerning clinical and supervisory interactions.

7.4 Ability to assist the supervisee in establishing and following policies and procedures to protect the confidentiality of clinical and supervisory records.

7.5 Ability to share information regarding documentation requirements of various accrediting and regulatory agencies and third-party funding sources.

8.0 **Task:** Interacting with the supervisee in planning, executing, and analyzing supervisory conferences.

**Competencies required:**

8.1 Ability to determine with the supervisee when a conference should be scheduled.

8.2 Ability to assist the supervisee in planning a supervisory conference agenda.

8.3 Ability to involve the supervisee in jointly establishing a conference agenda.

8.4 Ability to involve the supervisee in joint discussion of previously identified clinical or supervisory data or issues.

8.5 Ability to interact with the supervisee in a manner that facilitates the supervisee's self-exploration and problem solving.

8.6   Ability to adjust conference content based on the supervisee's level of training and experience.

8.7   Ability to encourage and maintain supervisee motivation for continuing self-growth.

8.8   Ability to assist the supervisee in making commitments for changes in clinical behavior.

8.9   Ability to involve the supervisee in ongoing analysis of supervisory interactions.

9.0   **Task:** Assisting the supervisee in evaluation of clinical performance

**Competencies required:**

9.1   Ability to assist the supervisee in the use of clinical evaluation tools.

9.2   Ability to assist the supervisee in the description and measurement of his/her progress and achievement.

9.3   Ability to assist the supervisee in developing skills of self-evaluation.

9.4   Ability to evaluate clinical skills with the supervisee for purposes of grade assignment, completion of Clinical Fellowship Year, professional advancement, and so on.

10.0   **Task:** Assisting the supervisee in developing skills of verbal reporting, writing, and editing.

**Competencies required:**

10.1   Ability to assist the supervisee in identifying appropriate information to be included in a verbal or written report.

10.2   Ability to assist the supervisee in presenting information in a logical, concise, and sequential manner.

10.3   Ability to assist the supervisee in using appropriate professional terminology and style in verbal and written reporting.

10.4   Ability to assist the supervisee in adapting verbal and written reports to the work environment and communication situation.

10.5   Ability to alter and edit a report as appropriate while preserving the supervisee's writing style.

11.0 **Task:** Sharing information regarding ethical, legal, regulatory, and reimbursement aspects of the profession.

**Competencies required:**

11.1 Ability to communicate to the supervisee knowledge of professional codes of ethics (e.g., ASHA, state licensing boards, and so on).

11.2 Ability to communicate to the supervisee an understanding of legal and regulatory documents and their impact on the practice of the profession (licensure, PL 94-142, Medicare, Medicaid, and so on).

11.3 Ability to communicate to the supervisee an understanding of reimbursement policies and procedures of the work setting.

11.4 Ability to communicate knowledge of supervisee rights and appeal procedures specific to the work setting.

12.0 **Task:** Modeling and facilitating professional conduct.

**Competencies required:**

12.1 Ability to assume responsibility.
12.2 Ability to analyze, evaluate, and modify own behavior.
12.3 Ability to demonstrate ethical and legal conduct.
12.4 Ability to meet and respect deadlines.
12.5 Ability to maintain professional protocols (respect for confidentiality, etc.).
12.6 Ability to provide current information regarding professional standards (PSB, ESB, licensure, teacher certification, etc.).
12.7 Ability to communicate information regarding fees, billing procedures, and third-party reimbursement.
12.8 Ability to demonstrate familiarity with professional issues.
12.9 Ability to demonstrate continued professional growth.

13.0 **Task:** Demonstrating research skills in the clinical or supervisory processes.

**Competencies required:**

13.1 Ability to read, interprets, and applies clinical and supervisory research.

13.2  Ability to formulate clinical or supervisory research questions.

13.3  Ability to investigate clinical or supervisory research questions.

13.4  Ability to support and refute clinical or supervisory research findings.

13.5  Ability to report results of clinical or supervisory research and disseminate as appropriate (e.g., in-service, conferences, publications)

# APPENDIX 11C
## SLP Assistant Suggested Competencies

I. Interpersonal Skills (communicates honestly, clearly, accurately, coherently, and concisely)

Deals effectively with attitudes and behaviors of the patient/client

Uses appropriate language (written and oral) in dealing with patient/client and others

Deals effectively with supervisor

II. Personal Qualities

Manages time effectively

Demonstrates appropriate conduct

III. Technical-Assistant Skills

Maintains a facilitating environment for assigned tasks

Uses time effectively

Selects, prepares, and presents materials effectively

Maintains documentation

Provides assistance to speech-language pathologist

IV. Screening

Demonstrates knowledge and use of a variety of screening tools and protocols

Demonstrates appropriate administration and scoring of screening tools

Manages screenings and documentation

---

*Note:* Abbreviated from "Speech-Language Pathology Assistant Suggested Competencies," ASHA 2006.

Communicates screening results and all supplemental information to supervisor

V. Treatment

Performs tasks as outlined and instructed by the supervisor

Demonstrates skills in managing behavior and treatment program

Demonstrates knowledge of treatment objectives and plan

# Chapter 12

# Leadership

*True leaders are not those who strive to be first, but those who are first to strive and give their all for the success of the team. True leaders are first to see the need, envision the plan, and empower the team for action. By the strength of the leader's commitment, the team is unleashed."*

(Anonymous)

## Introduction

Two terms that have many definitions are "professionalism" and "leadership." This chapter focuses on qualities of leaders and on models to gauge leadership styles with the learning styles of those being led. Day and Bobeva (2003) write that "Leadership may be construed as a state of mind, a process, a skill or a function: it can appear to be all these things and more." They go on to define the common factors for all the varied definitions of leadership as being the presence of a "leader and a set of activities performed by the leader, which creates and maintains a link to individuals, who are the followers of the leader" (p. 76). Any time you try to influence the behavior of another person, you are engaging in an act of leadership. Therefore, leadership can be defined as the process of influencing a group or an individual.

Leadership style is the pattern of behaviors you use when you are trying to influence others as perceived by them. Leadership style may fluctuate based on the setting and the tasks at hand. Your adopted leadership style for a particular task needs careful consideration if you want to develop your team and build motivational climates. "While your perceptions of your behavior are important, it tells you only how you 'intend' to act. It is helpful only if it matches the perceptions of those you are trying to influence." You may consider yourself to be "an empathetic, people oriented leader," but if your team thinks you are a "hard-nosed, task-oriented person," there is not a match between intent and perception, and this mismatch typically results in the team members feeling no allegiance to the leader (Junior League of Orlando-Winter Park, 1987). Keep in mind that without followers there are no leaders! As a leader, one should focus on developing positive relationships with those being led, as well as to focus on the task to be done.

**Task Block:** Think back over your life and review the leadership provided by peers, coworkers, family members, or anyone who is not a direct acquaintance (e.g., a politician or sports figure you have admired). What were the traits demonstrated by this individual that made him or her a good leader?

## Shared Governance

"Governance" refers to the participation of groups in a decision-making process. "Shared" can be thought of as "broad participation of diverse groups" (Gardiner, 2006, p. 62). Venable and Gardiner (1988) list six characteristics of shared governance:

1. climate of trust (integrity, consistency between words and deeds);
2. information sharing (disclosure of data necessary for decision-making);
3. meaningful participation (broad involvement in all aspects of decision-making and planning);
4. collective decision-making (moving toward group consensus);
5. protecting divergent views (valuing, nurturing alternative perspectives); and
6. redefining roles (all members are leaders) (Gardiner, 2006, p. 66).

The practice of shared governance implies that the decisions are not made by a single leader or manager, but by the collective will of all members of a leadership circle. It may be based on interactions of similar or diverse groups. Members of a leadership circle cooperate with each other and focus on the various possibilities to consider. "Circles promote life, discipline, and sacrifice for the common good" (Gardiner, p. 67).

## Climate of Trust

The first task of a team leader is to establish a bond of trust with the team members. In order to do this, the leader needs to emote confidence without cockiness, belief without doubt, and a basis of integrity to the mission of the team. If the team members have any doubt about the leader's true agenda and ability to lead, it is probable that no decision will be reached by the team, which will, in turn, frustrate and irritate the team members. So from the outset, the team leader needs to direct the team members toward functioning as a group to reach a common goal or solve a dilemma. Cartwright and Zander (1968), as cited by Day and Bobeva (2003), maintain that a leader must try to "satisfy both the goals of the group and the individual. The followers 'reward' the leader for this contract, by donating commitment, trust and ceding power-based status to the leader" (p. 77).

## Information Sharing

As team leader, it is expected that you will come to the table with data and concepts that need to be disclosed in order for the team to reach an informed and educated action plan and/or conclusion.

## Meaningful Participation

One of the cardinal issues when leading a team is to make each member of the team a critical component. A good team will have a leader who functions as a facilitator and sounding board, and will have members who all bring something different or unique to the table. Careful selection of a team can result in high productivity and group satisfaction if they are led in the proper manner. The leader of the team should make the team aware of the idea that the goal is not to win by making others lose in the decision-making process, but rather "it's a better way, a higher way" (Covey, 1989, p, 207).

### Collective Decision-Making

At the initial meeting, the leader needs to empower the team members by identifying tasks based on each individual's strengths. In addition, the leader needs to lead his followers in defining a vision, developing a mission statement, and determining goals that are meaningful to and achievable by the team members acting together (Gardiner, 2006).

### Protecting Divergent Views

We have all been in meetings where measured steps have been taken toward making a decision when someone speaks up and says, "Let me be the devil's advocate here." In my experience, these individuals are not out to sabotage the decision-making process; rather, they are presenting a different perspective that should be taken into consideration before making a final decision. There may be grounds for revising the decision that had not been part of the original discussion (Gardiner, 2006).

### Redefining Roles

When a decision has been reached, the group then should move toward developing an action plan. This is where a leader can capitalize on his or her observations of the team members up to this point. Strengths and weaknesses may have emerged that were unrecognized before. To this end, as decisions are reached regarding the steps of the implementation plan, the leader may challenge the members to redefine their roles "for the good of the team" (Gardiner, 2006).

## Are Management and Leadership the Same Thing?

Murphy (2000) wrote that "managers gain their power from the organization through a contractual arrangement, that is, a contractual arrangement between the organization and its workers. Leaders on the other hand draw their authority from the willingness of people to follow the leader." They frequently are used interchangeably, but the nature of the arrangement tends to lean toward having a dichotomy between the two. Murphy and Murphy (n.d.) maintain that when the workers are energized and involved with the project they are led, not just managed.

Stephen Covey (1989) writes the following:

> Management is a bottom line focus: How can I best accomplish certain things? Leadership deals with the top line: What are the things I want to accomplish: In the words of both Peter Drucker and Warren Bennis, "Management is doing things right; leadership is doing the right thing." Management is efficiency in climbing the ladder of success; leadership determines whether the ladder is leaning against the right wall. (p. 101)

Certainly there are projects when one may need to function as a manager and a leader; however, one must be careful about letting leadership become lost in the management demands.

## Leadership Behaviors

Some leadership behaviors may be characterized as mainly directing the followers'activities in terms of task accomplishment (*directive behavior*) whereas other leadership behaviors concentrate on providing social-emotional support and on building personal relationships between the leader and followers (*supportive behavior*). In still other situations, a combination of directive and supportive behaviors may be evident showing that leadership is not an either/or behavior. These patterns of behavior can be plotted on a grid using two separate axes. This results in four leadership styles.

Research shows that there is no "best" style of leadership. The style depends on the situation. Specifically, selecting the appropriate style means assessing:

1. The amount of direction (task behavior) needed.
2. The amount of social-emotional support (relationship behavior) needed.
3. The readiness or "maturity" of the follower to perform the objective.

In Situational Leadership, maturity or development level is defined as the competence and commitment of a follower to perform a specific task without supervision. The key is to determine the level of maturity and competence of those being led. The word "competence" is used rather than "ability" because people often use the word "ability" to mean potential. Competence can be developed with appropriate direction and support. It is a function of the leader to ensure that the knowledge and skills needed for a task can be gained from education, training, or experience.

Crosby (1996) lists four "leadership absolutes": a clear agenda, a personal philosophy, enduring relationships, and being worldly. Leaders who bring these attributes to the table will be more successful in eliciting commitment from their followers. Commitment is a combination of confidence and motivation. Confidence is a measure of a person's self-assuredness—feeling of being able to do a task well without much supervision. Motivation is a person's interest, willingness, and enthusiasm in doing a task. Crosby purports a leadership-personality grid (Table 12–1) based on five categories of leaders:

**Destructor:** Destructors tend to be insensitive to the will of his supervisees, and are typically appointed rather than elected to a leadership position. These self-centered individuals "are overbearing, aggressive people who are granted their own way in order to get them out of somebody else's office" (p. 10). Typically, they view things only from their own perspective with no regard for their coworkers.

**Procrastinator:** Procrastinators rarely work toward a goal. These individuals can rarely come to a conclusion that results in change. They are more comfortable with the status quo and waste the time and energy of fellow team members.

**Caretaker:** Crosby writes that these individuals are "frozen in time. Caretakers determine the best year they ever had and spend time trying to live it over again" (p. 18). It is not that they rebuke the idea of change; they just would prefer to rely on anything that worked in the past. They "avoid change, and establish a feeling of security and solidity" (Crosby, 1996, p. 25).

**Preparer:** A "preparer" also can be thought of as a learner and a planner. In the process of providing leadership, they focus on planned activities being implemented to achieve a common goal. They function in real time in a real world all while increasing their knowledge base. However, they would prefer "exploring the possibilities and laying the trail" (Crosby, 1996, p. 25).

**Table 12–1.** Leadership-Personality Grid

| | Destructor | Procrastinator | Caretaker | Preparer | Accomplisher |
|---|---|---|---|---|---|
| Agenda | "We'll do it this way now." | "I'll get back to you later on this." | "Make sure this doesn't violate any laws." | "Lay out the strategy so everyone can see it." | "We will review milestones each month." |
| Philosophy | "I know more than you do." | "Let's not rush things." | "If it isn't broken, don't fix it." | "I want us to be consistent in all things." | "I want everyone to know our philosophy." |
| Relationships | "I don't need anyone." | "Let's see how they work out first." | "We'll do what worked the last time." | "We need to have more seminars." | "Include customers, suppliers, and employees." |
| What we See: | Insensitive lout | Nervously reluctant | Frozen in time | Planned progress | Vibrantly consistent |

*Source:* From *The Absolutes of Leadership* by P. Crosby (1996). Copyright 1996 by Pfeiffer and Company. Reprinted with permission.

**Accomplisher:** A model of consistency, accomplishers are a complete package. "Relationships are successful, transactions are complete, strategies are well thought out and communicated, people are proud to be working with the accomplisher, and most business and personal interactions are successful" (pp. 23–24).

As interpreted by Brown and Barker (2001), "successful use of the Situational Leadership model relies on effectiveness in four communication components: communicating expectations, listening, delegating, and providing feedback." To that end, it is the responsibility of a leader to do the following tasks:

1. Create a vision with the followers (team players, partners, members, associates).
2. Facilitate and take action to assist the group in defining activities and goals to move toward the stated vision.
3. Help others develop commitment, skills, and behaviors that increase personal and organizational productivity toward reaching goals (http://preventiontraining.samhsa.gov).

Usually, those being led are at different levels on different tasks. Figure 12–1 illustrates these development levels. As a leader, one of your key jobs is to match your leadership style to the protégé's developmental level on that particular task. The leader should be focused on creatively guiding the worker to the self-actualization level (high competence and high commitment). According to this model, as the developmental level of individuals increases from D1 to D4, their competence and commitment fluctuates. When first beginning a new task where they have little or no prior knowledge or experience, most individuals are enthusiastic and ready to learn (D1). As they begin to perform the task, individuals often find it is either more difficult to learn or perform the task than they originally thought. This disillusionment decreases their commitment (D2). If they overcome this state and learn to perform the task with help from the leader, most people then go through a self-doubt stage where they question whether they can do the task well on their own. The leader says they are competent but they are not so sure. These alternating feelings of competence and self-doubt cause the variable commitment associated with D3—commitment that fluctuates from excitement to insecurity. With proper support, individuals can eventually become peak

| High Competence | High Competence | Some Competence | Low Competence |
|---|---|---|---|
| High Commitment | Variable Commitment | Low Commitment | High Commitment |
| **D4** | **D3** | **D2** | **D1** |

Developed ◄——————————————————————— Developing

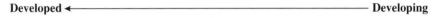

***Figure 12-1.*** This model identifies four developmental levels as illustrated. (From Junior League of Orlando-Winter Park (1989), *Seminar for Trainers*. Notes from seminar.)

performers who demonstrate high levels of competence, motivation, and confidence. In other words, given the appropriate amounts of direction and support, individuals move from one level of development to another, from being an enthusiastic beginner to a disillusioned learner to a reluctant contributor to a peak performer (Junior League of Orlando-Winter Park, 1987).

It is crucial to remember that someone's development level may be task-specific. They may be at the D4 level on one task and at the D2 level on another task. As a leader, one must recognize that different leadership styles are used for each task with a person to enhance his or her skill development—one size does not fit all with leadership.

## The Four Leadership Styles

Hersey, Blanchard, and Johnson (1996) developed a model of situational leadership in which the leaders assess the readiness level of their followers and adjust their leadership style accordingly. They developed a model (Figure 12-2) of leadership based on degrees of supportive leadership as opposed to directive leadership.

1.  Directing (high directive and low supportive) (Also called "TELLING").

    The leader defines the roles of the followers and tells them what, how, when, and where to do various tasks. Problem-solving and decision-making are initiated by the leader. Communication is largely one way, and implementation is closely supervised by the leader.

    People who need this style would see a leader who uses too much supportive behavior as permissive, easy, and rewarding poor performance. It is designed to assist people who do not have the skill or competence to do the required task.

2.  Coaching (high directive and high supportive) (Also called "SELLING").

    The leader provides a great deal of direction and leads with his or her ideas, but also attempts to hear the

| S3: Encourager: focus on minimizing direction on the task and increasing the relationships | S2: Coach: work on teaching the task as well as increasing the relationships with the led |
|---|---|
| S4: Delegator: decrease the amount of time spent on teaching the task as well as increasing the relationship. | S1: Structurer: primarily focus on teaching the task without working on the relationships |

| D4 | D3 | D2 | D1 |
|---|---|---|---|

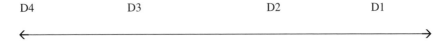

Developmental Level

**Figure 12–2.** Identifying the leader's activities in each of four styles of leadership. (Based on the work of Hersey and Blanchard, 1988.)

follower's feelings about decisions as well as their ideas and suggestions. Although two-way communication is increased, control over decision- making remains with the leader.

People who have started developing some competence but are unsure of their new skills respond better to the coaching style than to the directing style. It encourages followers to "buy into" the desired behaviors

3. Supporting (low directive and high supportive) (Also called "PARTICIPATION")

    The locus of control for day-to-day decision-making and problem-solving shifts from the leader to the follower with this style. The leader's role is to provide recognition and to actively listen and facilitate problem-solving/decision-making on the part of the follower. This style is appropriate when the follower has the ability to do the task.

4. Delegating (low directive and low supportive).

    The leader discusses problems with the follower until joint definition of the problem is reached. The decision-making process is then delegated to the follower. Note that it is the follower who has control over deciding how tasks are to be accomplished. Followers are allowed to "run their own show" as they have both competence and confidence to take responsibility

The developmental level is based on the person's willingness to do the job in addition to his or her ability to do the task (see Figure 12–2). Individuals at the D1 level typically have low competence but high commitment. Think about your first day at a new job. You are excited, anticipating success, and heavily invested in improving your performance. At the D2 level, there is some competence, but low commitment. This individual may be experiencing doubt about his abilities, which negatively affects his feeling of commitment. Workers at the D3 level of followers have high competence (they have been coached intensely in order to learn the task), and they are beginning to feel a resurgence of the commitment they had at the D1 level. Finally, at the D4 level, the employee has high competence, and high commitment. To use Maslow's term, these individuals have achieved self-actualization.

The S1 level should be used with new people. At this stage, it is critical that the leader give specific directions to accomplish the task. At the S2 level, the led may say, "You've told me what to do, but I'm not sure I'm ready." This person needs Style 2 supervision in which the leader stresses expresses belief in the employee by making statements such as, "You can do it."

Workers at the S3 level are sitting on the fence. In one breath, they will proclaim that they are ready, and then turn around and say, "I'm not really sure." As an encourager, the supervisor/leader needs to focus on building up a level of confidence in the employee. Finally, at the S4 level, the leader believes the employee is competent and confident; and is comfortable delegating tasks to him or her.

To determine the led's developmental level, it is helpful to start at the S4 level of leadership and see how the supervisee handles the task. After observing the supervisor in action, the leader can decide at what level he needs to provide guidance to the person taking on a new task. This is further explained in Table 12-2.

## Transformational Leadership

Transformational leadership is used frequently when leading a group of individuals in order to motivate them to realize their highest performance on the designated task. "Transformational leadership is inspirational leadership that gets people to do more while trying to achieve the highest performance" (http://atlas.kennesaw.edu/~ssavage1/case 2.htm; retrieved 07/06/07). Transforming leadership has been defined as "vision, planning, communication, or creative action, that has a positive unifying effect on a group of people around a set of clear values and beliefs, to accomplish a clear set of measurable goals" (http://prevention training.samhsa.gov). This approach has significant impact on the individual development of each person involved, as well as the organizational productivity of the group. As a leader of a group of individuals, one's job is to not only accomplish the established goals, but also to have a positive effect that unifies the individuals to be dedicated to the vision, beliefs, and values of the group.

Burns (1978) defines transformational leadership as a "relationship of mutual stimulation and elevation that converts followers into leaders and may convert leaders into moral agents" (p. 4). Through

**Table 12-2.** Hare's Cultural-Leader Role Extension to Hersey-Blanchard Instrument

| Leadership (Role) | Interactions (with Followers) | Affect (on Project) | Hersey-Blanchard Instrument Dimension |
|---|---|---|---|
| Worker-Leader | Competence, Power, Knowledge | Goal attainment | Task orientation |
| Personal-Leader | Trust, Friendship, Fidelity, Empathy | Team Integration | Relationship orientation |
| Cultural-Leader | Vision, Norms, Shared values | Contextual fit | Not covered at present |

*Source:* From "Successful IS Project Leaders: A Situational Theory Perspective" by J. Day & M. Bobeva in *Electronic Journal of Information Systems Evaluation*, *6*(2), p.83, 2003. Copyright: Academic Conferences Limited.

transformational leadership, the leader should focus on helping the members of the group to become better individuals. Bass (1990) writes that "The transformational leader asks followers to transcend their own self interests for the good of the group, organization, or society; to consider their longer term needs to develop themselves rather than their needs of the moment; and to become more aware of what is really important. Hence, followers are converted into leaders" (p. 53).

Leaders who practice transformational leadership empower their followers. "Instead of exercising power over people, transforming leaders champion and inspire followers. Tension can develop in this process. As leaders encourage followers to rise above narrow interests and work together for transcending goals, leaders can come into conflict with followers' rising sense of efficacy and purpose. Followers might outstrip leaders. They might become leaders themselves. That is what makes transforming leadership participatory and democratic" (Burns, 2003, p. 26).

## Transactional Leadership

"Transactional leadership, in which an exchange takes place between leader and follower, represents the traditional influence model found within most human groups" (Gardiner, 2006, p. 63). Typically, transactional leaders do not conform to the six criteria for shared governance as put forth by Venable and Gardiner (1988) (see page 264 of this chapter to review the six criteria). They exchange benefits with their followers, giving something to get something back in return from their followers. Transactional leadership refers back to the original concepts of leadership and, over the years, has proven to be the least productive in terms of leadership. Transactional methods frequently are employed by transformational leaders.

## Transcendent Leadership

In the late 1970s and early 1980s, a new type of leadership, transcendent leadership, evolved. Works by Greenleaf (1977), Bohm (1980), and Gandhi (2003) led to Diane Larkin's penning the term, "transcendent leadership." Gardiner writes that Larkin's (1995) concept of transcendent leadership is "to describe a special leadership she observed among leaders who transcend self into compassionate being and action" (p. 63). The transcendent leader has the "ability to lead from a consciousness of wholeness" (Gardiner, p. 64), modeled by Gandhi. The transcendent leader thinks reflectively, is value focused, facilitates dialogue, and is global in his or her perspective. Transcendent leaders help us more closely approach a world in which human's talents and energies are maximized, thereby improving all involved on personal, organizational, and global levels (Gardiner, 2006).

## Situational Leadership

Depending on the nature of the interaction, one may find him or herself switching from one leadership style to another. For example, in some situations, transactional leadership may be the leadership method of choice, whereas, in other situations, transformational leadership may be utilized. Situational leadership often melds translational and transformational leadership to improve group functioning as it progresses to realization of its goals as defined by a particular situation (Gardiner, 2006).

Gardiner bases the following statements on Hersey et al.'s definition of situational leadership:

> Hersey, Blanchard, and Johnson's (1996) use of situational leadership offered a good synthesis of the theory and practice of this pragmatic solution to dual leadership frames and is widely employed today by leadership scholars and practitioners. Hersey, Blanchard, and Johnson's emphasis on task and relationship—and the leader's use of each determined by situation—appealed to American pragmatists. (p. 63)

In 1938, in a discussion of situational leadership, Chester Barnard posited that leaders must strike a balance between the effectiveness (task) and efficiency (relationship). Nearly 65 years later, this balance is a critical component of situational leadership and in synch with the current American philosophy of pragmatism (Gardiner, 2006).

## Path-Goal Leadership

House (1971) defines the path-goal leadership theory as "one that clarifies paths through which followers can achieve both task-related and personal goals." There are four team leadership styles that comprise the path-goal leadership method:

1. directive leadership
2. supportive leadership
3. participative leadership
4. achievement-oriented leadership

Directive leadership of a team occurs when the team leader provides specific guidelines and instructions to the team members. This may include things such as clarifying expectations, assigning specific tasks, and laying general ground rules to be followed. Supportive leadership has been discussed previously in connection with the Hersey-Blanchard model of leadership. House explains supportive leadership as the leader's showing compassion, sensitivity, concern, and support for the followers. Through supportive leadership, it is hoped that a cooperative spirit among group members will be achieved.

Participative leadership focuses on needs of the situation, with the leader adapting his or her leadership style to one that best fits the needs of the situation at hand. All decision-making at this level is done by group consensus after everyone has shared their thoughts, ideas, and knowledge relevant to the task at hand. Day and Bobeva (2003) write that

> the most important ingredient defining the relationship between people in a project group is the nature and frequency of knowledge-based and affective interactions. The adaptive project leader is one who can dynamically and intuitively reconfigure the communications structures depending upon the exigencies of the project to meet speed, quality, stakeholder satisfaction, etc. (p. 83)

In achievement-oriented leadership, one establishes high goals, and then expects all involved to demonstrate their highest level of performance in the achievement of the established goals. It is also important that the leader demonstrate his utmost confidence in the group to achieve their goals.

## Summary

Good leadership is critical to the success of any team. This chapter has focused on the qualities of a leader as well as describing different models and styles of leadership. Day and Bobeva cite Edgmon (1995) in writing that successful "project leaders were adept at problem solving, giving of trust, recognizing achievement and coping with stress" (2003, p. 77). In closing, the following quote from Crosby (1996) sums up the information presented in this chapter:

> Systems integrity is when everything works as planned. It is the result of a carefully constructed, yet natural, operating culture. That culture cannot be purchased or packaged. It is a reflection of the leader's personal integrity. (p. 75)

# References

Barnard, C. (1938). *The functions of the executive*. Cambridge, MA: Harvard University Press.

Bass, B. M. (1990). *Bass & Stogdill's handbook of leadership: Theory, research, and managerial applications* (3rd ed.). New York: Free Press.

Bohm, D. (1980). *Wholeness and the implicate order*. London: Routledge & Kegan Paul.

Brown, N. A., & Barker, R. T. (2001). Analysis of the communication components found within the situational leadership model: Toward integration of communication and the model. *Journal of Technical Writing and Communication, 31*(2), 135–157.

Burns, J. M. (1978). *Leadership*. New York: Harper & Row.

Burns, J. M. (2003). *Transforming leadership: A new pursuit of happiness*. New York: Atlantic Monthly Press.

Cartwright, D., & Zander, A. (1968). *Group dynamics research and theory*. New York: Harper Row.

Covey, S. R. (1989). *The 7 habits of highly effective people: Powerful lessons in personal change*. New York: Free Press.

Crosby, P. B. (1996). *The absolutes of leadership*. San Diego, CA: Pfeiffer & Company.

Day, J. D., & Bobeva, M. (2003). Successful IS project leaders: A situational theory perspective. *Electronic Journal of Information Systems Evaluation, 6*(2), 75–86.

Gandhi, A. (2003). Leadership and nonviolence. In C. Cherry, J. J. Gardiner, & N. Huber (Eds.), *Building leadership bridges 2003* (pp. 1–11). College Park, MD: International Leadership Association & Center for Creative Leadership.

Gardiner, J. J. (2006). Transactional, transformational, and transcendent leadership: Metaphors mapping the evolution of the theory and practice of governance. *Leadership Review, 6*, 62–76.

Greenleaf, R. K. (1977). *Servant leadership*. New York: Paulist Press.

Hersey, P., & Blanchard, K. H. (1988). *Management of organizational behavior: Utilizing human resources* (5th ed.). Englewood Cliffs, NJ: Prentice-Hall.

Hersey, P., Blanchard, K. H., & Johnson, D. E. (1996). *Management of organizational behavior: Utilizing human resources* (7th ed.). Englewood Cliffs, NJ: Prentice-Hall.

House, R. (1971). A path-goal theory of leader effectiveness. *Administrative Science Leadership Review, 16*, 321–339.

Junior League of Orlando-Winter Park. (1987). *Seminar for trainers*. Notes from the seminar.

Larkin, D. (1995). *Beyond self to compassionate healer: Transcendent leadership*. Doctoral dissertation; Seattle University; 1995.

Murphy, R. M. (2000). *Strategic leadership vs. strategic management: Untying the Gordian knot.* Carlisle, PA: U.S. Army War College.

Murphy, R. M., & Murphy, K. M. (n.d.). *The lighted porch: The case for micro-leadership.* Unpublished manuscript.

Venable, W., & Gardiner, J. J. (1988, November 5). *Synergistic governance, leadership teams, and the academic department head.* Paper presented at the Annual Meeting of the Association for the Study of Higher Education, St. Louis, MO.

*Chapter 13*

# Time Management and Organizational Strategies

*When you kill time, you kill opportunities for success."*
Deep and Sussman (1995)

Smith (1997) writes that there are two sides to time management. One consists of those things that we want to do (e.g., increase our efficiency and effectiveness, spend more time with family), and the other side consists of those things we would like to avoid doing (e.g., being late to meetings, wasting time, forgetting obligations).

**Task Block 1:** List four things you wish to do, and four things you prefer to avoid doing.

In her writing about time management, Smith (1997) says there are two different kinds of time, and the most successful managers of time have developed an appreciation of the varieties of demands on their time. The two kinds of time are "the time that they must plan, control, and use in the most efficient way possible, and the time during which they can be free from the pressure of time" (Smith, p. 19). That being said, to be a good time manager, one must develop a constructive attitude about time by taking charge of one's life and taking responsibility for how one's time is used.

## The Paradox of Time

Time management is important at work because we are operating in a finite period. Leaving work undone can leave us frustrated at the end of the day and results in either carrying the task forward to another day, or working late. If we work late, fatigue may become an issue leading to a struggle to maintain the desired standard. These factors combined can produce a lower quality of work than we typically produce, thereby creating stress (Smith, 1997).

### *Question 1: What results occur when you leave work unfinished, and how does this make you feel?*

Smith (1997) warns that we need to avoid activity traps, one of which is the presence of activities that can act as barriers between an individual and his or her goals and objectives. When activities beyond one's control interfere with finishing a task and/or achieving personal goals and objectives, the stage is set for increased stress levels. In fact, it can become a vicious cycle because barriers to completing a task can create a crisis that needs managing, and crisis management, in and of itself, can lead to additional stress!

Working in a state of crisis management typically leads to making mistakes and, in general, performing poorly on the job. Smith (1997) suggests the following steps to resolve a state of crisis:

1. take "time out to consider the real purpose of your job, and what your priorities should be in relation to this purpose" (Smith, p. 15)
2. identify "the causes of those problems and involving others in finding long-term solutions to them" (Smith, p. 15) instead of dealing with problems as they occur
3. trust others which may require an investment of time in the beginning but will ultimately save time.

Another "activity trap" is being at everyone's beck and call (Smith, 1997). Compulsively looking after others fosters dependency in coworkers/supervisees instead of developing independent decision-making. Likewise, when a supervisee seems to be in over his or her head, the supervisor may be tempted to take over the task. This may save time in the short-run, but in reality, teaching the employee how to handle the task will save time for the employer in the long run. To resolve this activity trap, Smith suggests the following:

1. set limits on how much you are willing to get involved in solving problems other people are facing (p. 16)
2. give others responsibilities and teach them new skills so they can become more independent
3. offer support and guidance to others; do not take over their responsibilities and tasks

A third activity trap defined by Smith (1997) is being on a treadmill, or doing the same thing over and over. Not having variety in assignments and duties can lead to the development of feeling that one's talents are not being utilized adequately, and feelings that work-related tasks are not challenging enough to keep him or her interested in coming to work. This activity trap can lead to frustration, and frustration leads to stress in the workplace. One way to help resolve this particular trap is to sit down with your supervisor and/or supervisees and clarify "the purpose and responsibilities of your job" (Smith, p. 16).

To summarize Smith's (1997) concept of the "activity trap," it "means that we simply carry on doing things out of a misplaced sense of responsibility or out of habit. It means responding to a situation without thinking of the consequences of our actions" (p. 16). Breaking out of the activity trap requires that one focus on those goals he or she desires to achieve, set priorities and, then, decide how to use the time that is available most efficiently to achieve those goals in order of their priority.

## Personal Management

According to Butler and Hope (1995), personal management, not time management, is the issue. Good personal management results in good time management. According to them, the key principle of time management is "to spend your time doing those things you value or those things that help you achieve your goals." For example, if you are an altruistic person, you value spending time assisting others because one of your goals is to share your talents in helping others. Spend time doing what you value and what will help you reach your goals. If you only do the tasks that are the "most urgent," you will end up with distress and dissatisfaction.

Butler and Hope (1995) suggest an activity that is included here as Task Block 2. The point of Task Block 2 is not to think about your own death, but about the kind of person you want to be and the kinds of things you wish to achieve. The idea of thinking about this is to clarify what you would like them to say, not what you guess they would say. This statement will help you center your life around what you believe, not what others expect of you. It may change with time and circumstances, but the basic blueprint should be consistent across time.

**Task Block 2:** Imagine your own funeral three years from today. What would you *like* people to say about you? (Note: This is not the same as "What do I *think* they would say about me?") Based on your answer to this question, write a statement, for your own personal use, about your values and goals.

**How do you act in accordance with your values and goals?** We all probably will go through times when we may have to earn a living doing something we do not enjoy. It is sometimes helpful to rethink your plan of action in order to determine if there are alternative ways to reach our goal while honoring our values. To help you implement your plan, it is helpful to draw a **pie chart** indicating what percentage of time you will dedicate each week addressing your goals and values. The pie chart is further addressed in Task Block 3.

According to Butler and Hope (1995), the idea is that each of the activities that occupy your week can be classified in two ways: in terms of how ***important*** they are and how ***urgent*** they are" (p. 37).

Next, take your list of activities and tasks and list each one on a grid such as the one in Table 13–1.

The goal is not to spend time only on those things that are important, and more time on not urgent/important than on urgent/important. As you cut out the "not important" activities and tasks, spend more time engaging in "important/not urgent" activities. Develop a timetable to accomplish the tasks and activities. However, the timetable should not provide you with a rigid list of musts, but should be a helpful guide to make sure that, by and large, you spend your time following pursuits that fit with your goals and values (Butler & Hope, 1995).

**Table 13–1.** Task Classifications to Facilitate Time Management

| | |
|---|---|
| Urgent<br>Important | Not urgent<br>Important |
| Urgent<br>Not important | Not urgent<br>Not important |

A pie chart with an actual account of how you are spending your time can also be a helpful tool. How can you reconcile the differences between how you want to spend your time and how you actually spend your time?

Task Block 3 can take a bit of time to implement, but in the long run will provide valuable information that can be used to develop a time management program that helps you function in a more efficient and effective manner at work and at home.

**Task Block 3:** Keep a time diary for one week. Include the following information:

1. Note the activity/task, start time, finish time, and any comments.
2. Define life areas and determine the amount of time allocated to each one:
   a. Paid work
   b. Home and family
   c. Study time
   d. Unpaid work
   e. Leisure
   f. Maintenance (taking care of self, others, and your home)
   g. Sleep
3. Evaluate your data. Are the items that consume the most of your time in accordance with your goals and priorities? Develop a timetable that shows you where you are spending the bulk of your time.
4. Make a plan for how you are going to use your time based on the information you have gathered. Sometimes a pie chart such as Figure 13–1 can be used to indicate what percentage of time you will dedicate each week addressing your goals and values.

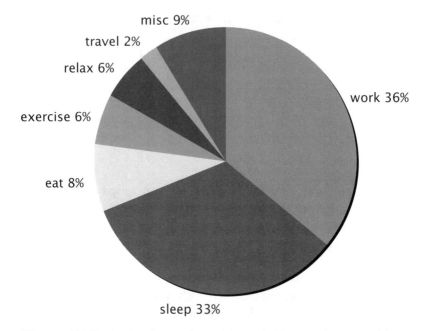

*Figure 13-1.* A pie chart of weekly activities such as working, sleeping, and eating, that can be used to indicate what percentage of time you will dedicate each week addressing your goals and values.

5. Develop a second timetable that can be used as a guide to make sure that you are spending your time to follow pursuits that fit with your goals and values.

## Three Main Ways That Time Gets Used Up

Many of us spend our lives dealing with crises and problems. To be an effective manager of time, one needs to plan ahead instead of constantly running from one crisis to another (Smith, 1997).

Often, we respond to the demands that others place on us. Sometimes, this is necessary in our work to "keep the boss happy." However, it frequently results in stress and losing sight of what we want to do with our lives (Smith, 1997). When this happens, it may be necessary to meet with the person who is placing the demands to discuss a timeline for completing the job without seriously compromising the tasks in which we are currently engaged. For example, when meeting with the "demander," one can say, "I'm currently engaged in this project, but I recognize the urgency of your request. If I stop what I am doing now to help you, could I have time set aside tomorrow to finish my task?"

As previously mentioned, Butler and Hope (1995) make the point that we will go through times when we may have to earn a living doing something we do not enjoy, or meeting the demands of others. When this happens, one may need to ask him or herself, "Given my current circumstances, are there other ways of achieving my goals?"

We do things out of habit, including dealing with crises and problems. Habits are routines, and repeated patterns of behavior. Having habits is not always bad; one just has to be sure that the habits he or she has are useful (Smith, 1997, p. 30).

## Nine Tools and Rules of the Time Management Trade

Butler and Hope (1995) have developed a list of rules and tools that can be used as mechanisms to manage time effectively.

1. Use your starter motor: Butler and Hope surveyed university students and found that the primary difference between average students and good students was in the ability of the student to settle down quickly to the task at hand. Frequently, we spend the time when we should be getting on with a task in limbo, meaning we do not start the task, but we do not enjoy our leisure time because we know the task awaits us.

2. Butler and Hope caution us not to let routine become our master. When used well, routine can release energy and time, not consume it. If one skips a routine once, then it is easier to skip it a second time, and it just does not get done (think about exercising).

3. Whenever we agree to do something more frequently than we should, the "yes" becomes a "no" to something else. Sometimes saying "Yes" leads to opportunities and unexpected treasures. "But the mistake most of us make is to say *yes* to too many things, so that we live according to the priorities of others rather than according to our own" (Butler & Hope, p. 40). You have to learn

to be assertive in saying *no* if the task will take away time from those things that are more important to your values and goals.

4. Distant elephants: At a distance, even large elephants look small. Similarly, a task that appears small and does not need to be done in the immediate time can take on a larger slice of our time if we say "yes" to too many requests made by others. Thus, if asked to complete an activity that is not important to you, no matter how long you have to complete the task, the task can take on the proportions of an elephant. The closer we get to the deadline, the larger the task becomes. Of course, sometimes saying "yes" leads to opportunities and unexpected joys. But, if we say "yes" too frequently, we begin to spend our time according to the priorities that others have instead of according to our own priorities.

5. Salami: Just as a butcher cuts a log of salami into smaller pieces, the salami principle holds that large tasks should be broken up into a series of small tasks. A small task is much less daunting than a large task. When faced with a large task, many of us never start them, or we start them but become disheartened and give up before we finish the task. Also, it is easier to predict how long it will take to do small tasks than one large one.

6. The Curse of Perfectionism: The time comes when there is not much to gain by putting in more effort. It is important to recognize when a task is done the best it is going to be, and to move on. For example, my daughter's first-grade teacher was a stickler for handwriting skills. In order to match her teacher's expectations, my daughter put in painstaking effort to have perfect handwriting. However, she put so much effort into being perfect with her script that she could not complete the task. The moral of the story is that perfectionism can result in slowness in completing a task and cause a task to be half-finished.

7. Once Past the Desk: Butler and Hope (1995) state that one should "either deal with the task straight away, or decide when to deal with it and put it aside until that time. The successful application of this technique requires a certain discipline. The discipline is made up of four steps, all of which should be taken with deliberation, at least until they become a habit" (p. 42). They posit that there are four steps to keeping items from piling up on the desk:

   a. Quick assessment of what you will need in order to deal with the matter

b. Decide when to tackle what you need to do

c. Put the matter aside until the allotted time

d. Carry out the action at the allotted time (p. 42).

Step 1 should be brief and be determined based on using your values as a yardstick. If the task is not important to you, do not undertake it. Step 2 is important if you need time to think about the task. Remember, thinking about a task and planning how to approach it are critical components of time management. Thus, there are some tasks that should be "mulled over" prior to taking action. As in step 1, the decision to set it aside temporarily should be a quick decision. Once the decision is made to set it aside, do so (step 3). When the allotted time for the task arrives, act decisively and carry out the task (step 4). Do not revisit the task without completing it.

8. Appointments need to end as well as start: Schedule the end of an appointment as well as the beginning so you will know when you are free for other appointments or activities. Furthermore, if all participants know when the meeting is scheduled to end, everyone will make better use of the time that has been allotted to the task.

9. Make time to plan: Periodically, review your priorities and proceed with whatever action plan works the best for you.

## Myths About Time Management

According to Smith (1997), one myth about time management is the belief that if you are efficient, you are also effective. In order to be efficient and effective, one must prioritize desired goals and objectives, and then do the things that are necessary to achieve those goals. *Webster's New Universal Unabridged Dictionary* (1997) defines "efficiency" as "accomplishment of or ability to accomplish a job with a minimum expenditure of time and effort," (p. 622) and it defines "effective" as "adequate to accomplish a purpose; producing the intended or expected result" (p. 622). An individual can be efficient in that he or she completes a task in a timely manner, but if the tasks he or she completes are not in concert with the overall goals of the work setting, he or she may not be regarded as being an effective employee.

**Task Block 4:** Identify someone whom you believe to be an efficient and effective individual. Ask him or her to tell you one method he or she uses as a time management strategy.

**Task Block 5:** Make a list of those attributes that you would use to describe an effective coworker.

A second myth identified by Smith (1997) is that there is "only one correct way to do a job" (p. 20). A mistake many managers make is to assume they know the best means for completing a task and to impose that means on the other employees. Supervisees are more likely to be good employees if they feel valued. The sense of being a valued employee is often based on the degree to which he or she is included in decision-making. When there is a job to be done, it is suggested that the employees meet together and answer the following questions that are proposed by Smith:

1. What is the purpose of the task?
2. What are the desired outcomes?
3. When should it be done?
4. Who should do it?
5. How should this task be done?

A third myth about time management is that in order to get good results, one has to put a lot of time into the task. Going back to myth #1, one needs to be efficient and effective. However, it is important to remember that it is the quality of the work, not the quantity of work that determines the effectiveness of the employee. An apparently efficient employee may complete many tasks in the course of the day, but do the tasks reflect quality work? Tasks done quickly could need time-consuming revisions that may hamper the work of others while waiting on those components of the task. Going back to the definitions of "efficient" as completing a task with minimal expenditure of time and effort, and "effective" as accomplishing a purpose, one can realize that just because an employee is efficient, he or she is not always effective. On the other hand, an employee may produce a quality product, but if he or she takes an inordinate amount of time to complete the task, this could slow down the ability of the team to accomplish their task in accordance with a predetermined deadline, (i.e., in an efficient manner).

Another myth is that in order for a job to be done well, one has to do it him or herself. Smith writes that "an inability or unwillingness to delegate is one of the primary causes of poor performance in business" (Smith, 1997, p. 20).

**Task Block 6:** Think about your fellow employees. Whom do you consider to be one that is particularly effective? Ask that person to describe his or her approach to a task.

A fourth myth is the belief that "you cannot be productive unless you are busy all the time" (Smith, 1997, p. 20). If one were to interview fellow employees, it is almost guaranteed one would find that efficient and effective employees take the time to think about a task carefully and plan a course of action to complete the task. Thinking time and planning time are essential components of time management. I spend the last 15 minutes of each workday planning the course of action to be taken on the following day. The tasks are listed in order with the most urgent being done first, and so on.

## Organization

In the discussion about time management, emphasis was put on establishing one's priorities, then assigning time schedules to complete those items. This strategy is applicable to organizational skills as well. Many people have indicated to the author that one of their best time management and organizational skills is making a daily and weekly list of what has to be done. "Organizing" is best implemented when priorities are written as action statements such as "Go to bank and set up college funds" as opposed to a phrase such as "children's education" (Davidson, 2004).

## Establishing One's Priorities

Davidson (2004) outlines a simple procedure that can assist in establishing one's priorities:

1. Write down everything that is important to you, assigned to you, or that you seek to achieve. Feel free to make this list long and involved.
2. Several hours later or even the next day, revisit your list. Cross out those things that, on second reading, are not that crucial. Combine any items that appear similar to each other. The object of this second encounter is to dramatically pare down your list. If you have too many priorities, you are likely to feel anxious and frustrated.
3. Now, restructure, redefine, and rewrite your list if necessary. Keep seeking to streamline it. When in doubt, toss it out. If you are not sure if an item belongs on the list, chances are it doesn't.
4. Put your list away and take it out the next day or the day after that. Now review it as if you are seeing it for the first time. Can any items be combined? Can anything be dropped? Should anything be reworded? As always, if something seems as if it is not that important, it probably isn't, so feel free to drop it!
5. Go ahead and make a working list of what you feel are your priorities at this time. Yes, things will shift and change as time marches on, but this is your list for now.

(A synopsis of this action procedure is in Chapter 9, Goal Setting, as it applies to both topics.)

## Reasons to Be Organized

One reason to be organized is to provide a safer environment. If one stores stacks of books on the floor, or a child has toys scattered about the room, there is an increased risk of someone's tripping and/or falling on the items.

A second reason to be organized is to be able to find items quickly and easily. When a colleague or student comes into our office space, we can be more responsive (and minimize the amount of time needed to meet) by having an organized office (Davidson, 2004).

A third reason is to increase the probability of making professional advances over time. If one were to look back at a list of employees who have been promoted and those who have not, one solid reason is the employee's organization skills. In this context, organization means more than having a neat office with all critical elements easily accessed. An organized person is usually an expert at delegation. This could include the development of flow charts and/or lists explaining the role everyone has in completing a project. This does not have to be at the office alone. These strategies are helpful in the home setting as well.

Before beginning to organize, for example, your desk, ask yourself the following questions:

What will be involved?

What kind of energy will I lend to the assignment?

What will I do first?

How will I take charge?

How will I feel when the task is completed? (Davidson, p. 46)

## What Do the Best Time Managers Do?

According to Smith (1997), the best managers of time are those individuals who have "developed a sense of different kinds of time" (p. 18). There is the time that must be planned, controlled, and used as efficiently as possible, and there are the times that they can "be free from the pressure of time" (Smith, p. 18). In other words, one must learn to relax and enjoy unscheduled time in addition to our well-planned and thought-out schedules in order to be satisfied with life. Smith encourages us to develop a constructive attitude about time by taking control of our lives and being responsible for how we use our time.

## Strategies Used by Practicing Speech-Language Pathologists

As part of the preparation for writing this chapter, the author conducted a survey of practicing speech-language pathologists about the time management and organizational strategies they employ. Lists of these strategies are in Tables 13–2 (time management) and 13–3 (organizational strategies).

**Table 13–2.** Time Management Strategies Used by SLPs

**Hospital-Affiliated Outpatient Clinic**

Utilizing time between patients to complete note writing

Prioritizing

Staying on top of paperwork

Maintaining organized strategies

Keeping organized with a schedule

Do not handle your mail twice

Begin writing daily notes when patient is given a break in therapy

**Acute-Care Hospitals**

When I have open gaps/cancellations, I block that time for paperwork

Keep paperwork efficient, yet exact, to meet required documentation

When possible, do reports immediately after diagnosis/ treatment sessions

Prioritizing

**University Clinics**

Reading E-mails in bulk at preset times (every 2 hours)

Getting to work early

Multitasking/doing paperwork as soon as submitted

Making sure I schedule blocks of time to catch up on paperwork

Holding meetings on time

Complete everything on daily list

Never delay (stay on top of things in order to deal with interruptions)

**Table 13–2.** *continued*

Making lists and checking off completed items

Do routine tasks first and get them off my desk

Prioritizing (but my priorities do not always reflect those of my administrators)

Complete short administrative tasks in between patient sessions

Making lists with timelines

**Skilled Nursing Facility**

Making a schedule at the beginning of the day

**Elementary Schools**

Keeping organized as much as possible

Keeping needed forms/materials readily available

Making lists of priorities

**Private Practices**

Get to work before everyone else and work in the quiet time before the storm

Have an idea of what activities I want to do with each patient a day ahead of time

Allowing time to discuss therapy/evaluation with caregivers and answer their questions

**Community Clinics**

Becoming more of a clock watcher

Expecting more from my patient when not in therapy

Making a list of what needs to be done by priority so the "Have to" tasks get done

**Table 13–3.** Organizational Strategies Used by SLPs

**Hospital-Affiliated Outpatient Clinic**

Preparing early in the work day

Writing notes

Prioritizing

Maintaining a schedule with allotted paperwork time

Keeping organized with a schedule

Delegating

Completing all paperwork each day

Not leaving work for tomorrow

Staying on top of your work

Finishing morning work before the afternoon work begins

**Acute-Care Hospitals**

Having files created for paperwork/forms

Using a daily planner of my own (separate from the master schedule)

Factoring in phone calls, meetings, and paperwork time

Allowing for 30 minutes of unexpected interruptions on the schedule

Prioritizing

Writing notes

**University Clinics**

Using a yearly visual planner and developing procedural flowcharts

Making a "to do" list

Outlining tasks/check off systems and deadlines

Computerizing information as much as possible so I can easily retrieve and revise files

Making a list at home for the next day at work

Using a daily/weekly/monthly planner

**Table 13–2.** *continued*

"Batching" tasks (set aside time in weekly planner for phone calls, paperwork, etc.)

Closing my office door during "crunch" times

Making appointments with students to cut down on interruptions

Adhering to a calendar

Setting up methods/procedures of organization and sticking to them

**Skilled Nursing Facilities**

Keeping daily records

Sorting files

**Elementary Schools**

Use a fairly detailed filing system that allows for quick storage and retrieval

Making a prioritized list of things to be done

Prioritizing my piles

**Private Practices**

Never touching anything twice

Dealing with things as soon as possible

Keeping all patient materials in the patient's folders.

Organizing all patient folders in the same way to facilitate access to needed information

Keeping patient goals/treatment plans at front of each patient's folder

**Community Clinics**

Making lists

Preplanning tasks and sticking to the plan

Keeping up with filing

Documenting patient contact hours on a daily basis rather than waiting for it to pile up

## Summary

Smith encourages us to make realistic decisions to use our time effectively and efficiently in order to achieve our goals in life. Specifically, one critical aspect goes back to the presented idea of "personal management," not just "time management." We have to be aware of our goals in order to facilitate decision making, then to decide how much time we will give to each demand on our time. We should learn productive habits. "Being better at managing our time means making sure that we decide how we are going to use our time—and that these decisions get us closer to achieving our goals" (Smith, 1997, p. 30).

## References

Butler, G., & Hope, T. (1995). *Managing your mind: The mental fitness guide.* New York: Oxford Press.

Davidson, J. (2004). *The 60 second organizer: Sixty solid techniques for beating chaos at home and at work.* Avon, MA: Adams Media.

Deep, S., & Sussman, L. (1990). *Twenty-one ways to make time your slave.* Reading, MA: Addison-Wesley.

Smith, J. (1997). *How to be a better time manager.* London, UK: The Industrial Society.

Waitley, D. (1997). *The new dynamics of goal setting: Flextactics for a fast changing future.* New York: William Morrow.

Webster, N. (2003). *Webster's new universal unabridged dictionary.* New York: Barnes & Noble.

## APPENDIX 13A
## Twenty-One Ways to Make Time Your Slave*

1. Record in one calendar-planning system . . . all the projects and people you manage. Write down in the action section every commitment you make at the time you make it, and then transfer the commitment to the date in your calendar when it will come due. Put your daily 'to do' list on the first page in that planner, and change it every day.

2. "Plan each week the week before, and plan each day the day before.

3. "Stop wasting the first hour of your workday.

4. "Do one thing at a time, and do it well. It takes time to start and stop work on each activity. Stay with a project until it is completed.

5. "Create a time-analysis chart of your activities. Break your day into fifteen-minute blocks. Note your chief activity or activities for each block. After logging your activities for a week or so, you'll have a representative sample of how your time is spent. Study the results. Decide what you can do to make better use of your time.

6. "Establish time limits for meetings and conversations in advance. Consult your watch when a deadline approaches. End the conversation when it arrives. Wristwatch alarms or beepers can be effective tools in keeping meetings within limits.

7. "Don't open unimportant junk mail. At least 25% of the mail you receive can be thrown away without taking the time to open it.

8. "Try to handle each piece of paper only once—including faxes, letters, and memos—and never more than twice. Do not set anything aside without taking some action. Some executives carry briefcases full of faxes, letters, and memos around for days without taking action. By the time they act, they are often too late to capitalize on the opportunity. For you as a 21st century achiever one computer disk for a notebook computer is better than a steamer trunk full of papers.

---

*Reprinted from *The New Dynamics of Goal Setting: Flextactics for a Fast Changing Future* by D. Waitley. Copyright, 1997 by William Morrow Company, an Imprint of Harper Collins, New York, NY. Reprinted with permission.

9. "Carry work, reading material, audiotapes, and your laptop computer with you everywhere you go. Convert downtime into uplink time.

10. "Write answers in the margins of letters you receive and mail or fax the letter back to the sender.

11. "Recognize when your peak energy occurs during the day. Allocate the most difficult projects to that period. Work on easy projects at low-energy times.

12. "When you feel that your energy level is dropping, take a break. For many people, this occurs around 3:00 in the afternoon. For you, it may be in the early morning or right after lunch.

13. "Get enough rest, nutrients, and exercise. If you don't feel well, you can't do well. Maintain your health and build your stamina. Treat your body the way you would if it were a space shuttle you were about to be launched in. Treat yourself as if you are worth the effort and expense it takes to nurture yourself!

14. "Set aside personal relaxation time during the day. Don't work during lunch. It's neither noble or nutritional to skip important energy-input and stress-relieving times.

15. "Take shorter vacations more often and leave your work at home. The harder you work, the more you need to balance your exercise and your leisure time.

16. "When possible, plan your work so your projects end when your day does. Take work home only as an exception, not the rule. Your professional life needs a whole human being, one with a satisfying personal life.

17. "End the day by listing all tomorrow's important priorities. Incorporate these projects into your daily 'to do' list.

18. "Throughout the day, ask yourself, 'What's the best use of my time right now?' As the day grows short, focus on projects you can least afford to leave undone.

19. "Each day, take some time to focus on your long-term dreams. You will keep your motivation vivid and strong. I take a walk of at least 15 minutes every day, rain, snow, or shine. If the weather is bad, I walk through an indoor mall. While I am walking and exer-

cising, I think about my life goals. It's a great way to window-shop, and if I keep walking it saves money too!

20. "(You may not get too excited about this suggestion, but it has worked wonders for me!) Consider getting up 40 minutes earlier in the morning and going to bed 40 minutes earlier. You may need to inch into this habit by setting your alarm 10 minutes earlier each week for four weeks. The extra 40 minutes in the morning can become some of your most productive, personally rewarding, 'home alone' time. Use the 40 minutes to think about what is really important for you to accomplish with this full day ahead of you. By going to bed 40 minutes earlier, you may have to sacrifice a few one-liners by Jay Leno or David Letterman, but they won't mind, and after all, they are well on their way to reaching their life goals, while not the least bit concerned with your reaching yours.

21. "Make certain your television set is in a cabinet that has a door on it that you can close. Treat it as it deserves to be treated. It is just one of your appliances, not your trusted armchair or bedside companion. The average American adult spends about 30 hours per week in a TV-induced stupor. Children spend even more time this way, which is why they are out of shape and also why they are staying home longer after they graduate from high school and college. They are used to tension-relieving activities, rather than goal-achieving actions." (p. 91).

# Chapter 14

# Group Dynamics

Over the course of one's professional life, speech-language pathologists will be members of and/or interact with a variety of types of groups. There are a variety of different kinds of groups as delineated by Molyneaux and Lane. Specifically, Molyneaux and Lane (1990) list these types of groups:

1. groups of clients—typically with similar problems or common therapy objectives
2. groups of family members of clients with communication disorders
3. groups composed of professionals from various disciplines, such as a cleft palate panel or other diagnostic team
4. groups composed of professionals and a client and family members meeting together to plan a client's educational program or an appropriate educational or agency placement
5. continuing education or college classes in which the professional may be either student or instructor
6. committees functioning as part of professional or other organizations of which the clinician is a member
7. other groups in which the professional is interested and takes part; for example, as a community service or as a recreational activity (p. 119).

Molyneaux and Lane (1990) go on to say that one classification of a group is based on the primary purpose of the group. A second type of group is one that is defined by a characteristic that all members have, such as the American Speech-Language-Hearing Association.

A third manner is the defining a group as being formal or informal. Table 14–1 delineates the differences of these two types of groups. Examples of formal groups are standing committees, task forces, advisory

**Table 14–1.** Formal and Informal Group Functioning

| Formal Group | Informal Group |
|---|---|
| Persons have titles and positions; there is a designated leader | Roles emerge and shift; there is no designated leader |
| There are written rules and procedures. | There is improvised and casual conversation. |
| New members receive specific training or indoctrination | What informal training there is occurs in the course of group meetings. |
| There are written agendas and meetings. | Members sometimes take notes; people often rely on memory. |
| Meetings are scheduled. | Meetings occur as needed or as people are available. |
| Members are specialists. | Members are generalists. |
| Decision-making occurs by voting or referral to a higher authority. | Decision making occurs by consensus. |

*Source:* From *Effective Group Communication* (p. 65) by E. Stech and S. A. Ratliffe, 1985, Lincolnwood, IL: National Textbook Company. Copyright 1985 by National Textbook Company. Reprinted by permission.

boards, boards of directors, project groups, management teams, and law-making groups. Informal groups "are composed of individuals who come together in an impromptu fashion to talk over problems or issues or who are temporarily drawn together because of an immediate interest or task" (Molyneaux & Lane, 1990, p. 122). Sometimes, a group will adopt aspects of both types of group. Table 14–1 demonstrates the differences between a formal group and an informal group.

As cited in Molyneaux and Lane, Combs, Avila, and Purkey (1978) described four types of groups in which individuals in the helping professions participate:

1. conversation groups, characterized by casual interaction of members in a social manner; instruction groups, designed to show or tell participants something;
2. instruction groups, designed to show or tell participants something;
3. decision groups, formed to arrive at a decision or consensus on some matter; and
4. discovery groups, designed to aid participants in gaining new insights into their own behavior and their relationships with others (p. 123).

## Stages of Developing a Group

Tuckman (1965), as cited by Molyneaux and Lane (1990), posits that there are four stages in the development of a group: forming, storming, norming, and performing. In the forming stage, the members get to know each other, define the task at hand, and clarify that all members have a role. Then, in the storming stage, members compete with each other to determine who will be the leaders of the group, and wrestle with how the group will function, what the group's missions should be, and actions the group needs to take. In the norming stage, the members start to feel an allegiance to the group, and they develop the rules and operational procedures of the group. At the end of the norming stage, the members "gel" into a well-defined group. Finally, in the performing stage, the group members focus on the tasks to be accomplished and take steps in those directions.

According to Shulman (1979), the making of a group follows an evolutionary pattern.

> The group must go through a developmental process just as any other growing entity. Early tasks include problems of formation and the satisfaction of individual members' needs. Problems of dealing with the worker as a symbol of authority (authority theme) must be faced, as well as the difficulties involved in peer-group relationships (the intimacy theme). Attention needs to be paid to the culture of the group so that norms which are consistent with the achievement of the group's goals are developed. Taboos that block the group must be challenged

and mastered if the discussion is to be meaningful. Finally, a formal or informal structure must be developed. This structure will include assigned roles, assigned status, communication patterns, and a decision-making process. Effective work in the group will develop a sense of cohesion that, in turn, will strengthen future work. (pp. 257–258)

## Facilitative Communication Behaviors

An unknown source has identified eight communication behaviors that facilitate communication in a group. These are discussed as follows:

1. Summarizing: Summarizing is a useful tool when monitoring group interactions. To hold miscommunications at bay, the summarizer will recap the essence of what the speaker has to say.
2. Compromising: Compromising is defined in *Webster's New Universal Unabridged Dictionary* (1996) as "a settlement of differences by mutual concessions; an agreement reached by adjusting of conflicting or opposing claims, principles, etc. by reciprocal modification of demands" (p. 42). Some groups will require that someone assume the role of mediator. This is particularly true when there is a divide among the group members that blocks the road to a decision.
3. Encouraging: Many groups need a "cheerleader" who encourages the group through working together toward a common cause. At times, it is possible that, if someone is too "gung-ho," their comments could be annoying. However, it behooves all group members to realize that this individual has the best interests of the group in mind.
4. Proposing actions/options: This individual falls into the description of a group member who suggests possible actions, options, and solutions.
5. Analyzing actions/options: The analyzer breaks the big issue into smaller bits and proposes actions and/or options for the group to consider as it moves through the process of making a decision.
6. Organizing information: The organizer in a group is the one who takes notes, and groups related bits of information into an outline, with the ultimate goal of leading the group to a decision.

7. Sharing information: It is imperative when a group is making a decision as a team that all information be "laid on the table." If a group member withholds information that is germane to the matter at hand, reaching a consensus can be harmed. Thus, everyone in the group should be willing to share any information he or she has with regard to the issue at hand.
8. Being aware of patterns of communication (Who talked? How long? To whom? Did a leader emerge? Why or why not?)

**Task Block 1:** List three characteristics of the people that you interact with *most* efficiently.

## Behaviors That Hinder Communication

The same unknown source also developed a list of communication behaviors that are a hindrance to communication:

1. Withholding information: Team members need to be on "the same page" when it comes to making a group-based decision. The work of the team can be destroyed if there are team member(s) who deliberately withhold information that could have an influence on the team's decision-making process. When information is minimal the definition of the problem will be inadequate. Great emphasis must be placed on fact finding if a group is to solve a problem effectively.
2. Poor communication: When poor communication occurs within the group, and particularly with the leader, team members may have a lack of information. Poor communication can result in a lack of clarity in stating the problem. Much of the initial effort of groups is directed toward orienting members to what the problem is. Remember, effective communication is needed to have effective problem-solving.
3. Premature decision: Formulating a decision before all information has been obtained can result in an incomplete or inaccurate decision. Groups should create an atmosphere that supports the presentation and the pooling of a wide assortment of ideas.
4. Not organizing information: Sometimes when one is making a decision, he or she has a haphazard system of information, not

easily being able to access all the information he or she has, resulting, again, in an incomplete or inaccurate decision.

5.  Not sharing information: Some individuals, often for reasons known only to themselves, will withhold information that may have an impact on the group's ability to achieve its purpose and/or goals. The leader needs to impart to every team member that withholding information can be injurious to the process.

6.  Pressures for conformity: This slows the development of different ideas. Divergent thinking as well as convergent thinking is necessary for sound problem-solving.

7.  Lack of inquiry and problem-solving skills: Some groups may need special training in how to use these methods to their advantage.

8.  Inadequate motivation: Any problem-solving group must be motivated to solve its problems. Members who leave work to others clearly lack motivation.

**Task Block 2:** List three characteristics of the people that you interact with *least* efficiently.

**Task Block 3:** List three personal needs that you must have satisfied in order to be motivated and committed in your work environment.

## Group Roles

As groups develop, the inclination is for the members to choose different roles, whether it be a conscious decision or the result of evolution of the group. Napier and Gershenfeld (1985) described the different types of roles that are typically represented in a group.

### Work Roles

Work, or task, roles are those that facilitate getting the job done.

1.  ***Initiator-Informer:*** Proposing tasks, goals, actions; defining group problems; suggesting procedures; offering facts; giving an opinion.

2. ***Clarifier-Summarizer:*** Interpreting ideas or suggestions; defining terms; clarifying issues before the group; pulling together related ideas; offering a decision or conclusion for the group to consider.
3. ***Reality Tester:*** Testing an idea against some data trying to see if the idea would work

## Group Building and Maintenance Roles

Group building and maintenance roles are those that facilitate membership in the group.

1. ***Harmonizer-Compromiser:*** Mediating; conciliating differences in points of view; making compromise solutions; modifying in interest of group cohesion or growth.
2. ***Gate-Keeper-Encourager:*** Helping to keep communication channels open; facilitating the participation of others; being friendly, warm and responsive to others; praising others and their ideas; agreeing with and accepting contributions of others.
3. ***Consensus Tester:*** Asking to see if a group is nearing a decision; sending up "trial balloons" to test group opinions.

## Egocentric Roles

Egocentric roles are roles that serve the individual's needs, not the groups' needs. It may be necessary to set norms for the group in an effort to control those who assume self-oriented roles. Examples of norms would be: (1) all members agree to abide by the consensus; (2) do not express opinions that are based solely on personal opinion; and if one does express an opinion based on personal issues, state that (3) those who are unable to abide by the consensus should disqualify themselves.

1. ***Blocker:*** Disagreeing and opposing beyond "reason" = resisting the group's wish for personally oriented reasons; using hidden agenda to thwart the movement of a group.
2. ***Aggressor-Dominator:*** Deflating status of others; attacking the group or its values; asserting authority or superiority to manipulate

group or certain members; interrupting contributions of others; controlling by means of flattery or other patronizing behavior.

3. *Playgirl-Avoider:* Making a display in "playgirl" fashion of one's lack of involvement; horsing around; seeking recognition in ways not relevant to group task. Pursuing special interests not related to the task; staying off subject to avoid commitment; preventing group from facing up to controversy (Junior League of Orlando-Winter Park, 1987; Molyneaux & Lane, 1990; Napier & Gershenfeld, 1985).

## Suggestions for Conducting Small Group Discussions

Every meeting of the group should have an introduction/beginning, an elaboration (middle), and concluding (closing) phase.

1. One may initiate a discussion by stating a problem, by asking open-ended questions, or by beginning with a controversy. Invite the members of the group to speculate and allow them to play with ideas.
2. What is the goal? Goals are needed to learn about the subject, to solve a problem, and to discuss an issue. Have group members write down goals and problem solutions, and then share them with the group.
3. Moving into the elaboration phase, the leader should talk less and listen more. This will facilitate group discussion.
4. In the closing phase, the leader and/or "summarizer" should recap the important issues brought up in the elaboration phase and lead the group through the discussion designed to facilitate the decision-making.
5. Rotate the role of leader.

## Team Task Analysis

It is a good idea periodically to conduct an analysis of the team's efforts. Questions to be addressed in this process include the following:

1. What are our strengths as a team?
2. What are our weaknesses as a team?
3. How can each member contribute to the problem-solving process? Along these lines, it is a good idea to refer to the roles of team members described earlier in this chapter to see who fits into each role.

## Summary

Groups are formed for a variety of reasons and to meet a variety of needs. It is important for group members to be familiar with the various roles that group members can assume, and how each of those roles affects both the cohesion of the group, and the ability of the group to address identified issues. Being a member of a group comes with designated issues and problems to discuss with others and, hopefully, provide resolution that is satisfactory to all involved.

**Acknowledgments.** Personal notes from leadership training workshops served as a foundation for this chapter. The author would like to thank all those who have offered these workshops in the past.

## References

Junior League of Orlando-Winter Park, FL, Inc. (1987). Fall Trainer's Seminar.

Molyneaux, D., & Lane, V. W. (1990). *Successful interactive skills for speech-language pathologists and audiologists*. Rockville, MD: Aspen.

Napier, R. W., & Gershenfeld, M. K. (1985). *Groups: Theory and experience* (3rd ed.). Boston: Houghton Mifflin.

Shulman, L. (1979). *The skills of helping individuals and groups*. Itasca, IL: F. E. Peacock.

Stech, E., & Ratliffe, S. A. (1985). *Effective group communication*. Lincolnwood, IL: National Textbook.

*Webster's New Universal Unabridged Dictionary*. (2003). New York: Barnes & Noble Books.

# Chapter 15

# Professionalism and Conflict of Interest

## Professionalism Defined

Cruess, Johnston, and Cruess (2004, p. 74) define a profession as follows:

> An occupation whose core element is work based upon the mastery of a complex body of knowledge and skills. It is a vocation in which knowledge of some department of science or learning or the practice of an art founded upon it is used in the service of others. Its members are governed by codes of ethics and profess a commitment to competence, integrity and morality, altruism, and the promotion of the public good within their domain. These commitments form the basis of a social contract between a profession and society, which in return grants the profession a monopoly over the use of its knowledge base, the right to considerable autonomy in practice and the privilege of self-regulation. Professions and their members are accountable to those served and to society.

A distinguishing characteristic of professionalism is "the expectation that a professional will subordinate self-interest" (Swick, 2000, p. 612) and maintain an altruistic attitude toward those who have health care needs. Given the numerous people and agencies to which a professional must answer, it is inevitable that conflicts of interest may arise. Some of these people and agencies include the scope of practice, certification standards and Code of Ethics of the American Speech-Language-Hearing Association (ASHA), policies and procedures for the work site, demands and expectations from immediate boss, our patients, our coworkers, third-party payer regulations, and federal and state legal mandates.

Medical and allied health professionals must be committed to academic integrity, and to being a lifelong learner. Swick (2000, p. 613) writes that "a commitment to excellence makes life-long learning fundamental to professionalism." Health care professionals must demonstrate "the capacity to recognize and accept limitations in one's knowledge and clinical skills, and a commitment to continuously improve one's knowledge and ability." (AAMC, 1998, p. 5) As a clinical educator, I stress to my students that their diploma does not mean that education is over—that it needs to continue throughout their professional life, and sometimes, beyond. Recently, I had a gentleman who looked to be in his 70s sit in on my class. He was conversing with a student next to him, so I assumed they knew one another and I asked the student to introduce him. She told us his name and said he was just sitting in on the class. After class he approached me and identified himself as a former professor at the University of Florida who had retired and cared for his ill wife. After his wife died, he decided to resume his dedication to learning. Thus, he would roam the halls of a large classroom building and talk to the students about what they were learning. If it sounded interesting to him, he would sit in on that class. What a shining example he was for our students! He returned to my class a few more times. After a lecture on aphasia, he told me his wife had suffered with aphasia and heart ailments, and it was nice to see that "our young people" were being educated about this subject in the event that one of their loved ones fell prey to aphasia, and so they would be prepared to help people such as his wife.

Professionals must respond to societal demands and needs, essentially having a "social contract" with their community. In order to best meet its obligations, any professional must actively address the societal needs of his or her community. This is a critical component in preventing deficits that negatively affect speech, language, and hearing. Almost by definition, any individual involved in a health care profession such as speech-language pathology is going to face issues and reflections on moral values that will cause us to behave and accomplish our many duties in an ethical manner. This includes our interactions with our patients, as well as with our community and societies. This may include such things as setting up a sliding scale and/or getting grant support to provide diagnostic and treatment services to the indigent and underserved populations in one's community (Swick, 2000).

Such humanism is considered by some to be a critical component of professionalism; others do not see it in that manner. Swick (2000) maintains that health care providers demonstrate the qualities of "core humanistic values, including honesty and integrity, caring and compassion, altruism and empathy, respect for others, and trustworthiness" (p. 612). It is hard to believe that any health care professional would not demonstrate these humanistic values as the patients are the focus of our attention and ministrations.

Wynia, Latham, Kao, Berg, and Emmanuel (1999) maintain that there are three core elements of professionalism.

> First, professionalism requires a **moral commitment** to the ethic of medical service which we will call devotion to medical service and its values. This devotion leads naturally to a **public, normative act**: public profession of this ethic. Public profession of the ethic serves both to maintain professional's devotion to medical service and to assert its values in societal discussions. These discussions lead naturally to **engagement in a political process of negotiation**, in which professionals advocate for health care values in the context of other important competing societal values. (p. 1612)

"Professional work has always been, at its best, a collegial endeavor rather than an entrepreneurial enterprise" (Swick, 2000, p. 613). However, an addendum to this statement is that the health care professions need to maintain accountability in order to earn autonomy.

## Authority

Sociologist Max Weber defined three types of authority: (1) legal authority in which commands are obeyed because the people recognize them as legally legitimate coming from a legal authority; (2) traditional authority whereby people follow your commands because it is what they have always done, and (3) charismatic authority in which people follow your commands because "something in your personality compels their obedience" (Latham, 2002, p. 364). When Talcott Parsons, also a sociologist, translated Weber's work into English, he believed a fourth type of authority should be added to Weber's list: legitimate authority. Parsons also called this "expert authority" in which individuals obey your commands because "they believe that you know something they do not know" (Latham, 2002, p. 364). Parsons maintains that legitimate authority is associated with interactions with professionals, and that professionals "are therefore constantly invoking their authority to negotiate and re-negotiate the normative boundaries between individuals and society" (Latham, 2002, p. 364). For example, a speech-language pathologist may recommend that a patient with a weak voice employ a voice amplifier thus enabling her to return to her profession of classroom teaching in an elementary school.

Latham (2002) makes the point that "one has authority if one's statements give others new and sufficient reason for holding a belief or taking an action" (p. 365).

## Autonomy and Accountability

Health care professionals "exercise accountability for themselves and for their colleagues. Implicit in relative autonomy granted to a profession is that its members will set and enforce standards of practice. Demonstrating true accountability is key to maintaining the privilege of autonomy"(Swick, 2000, p. 612) that, for many decades, has been held close by medical practitioners. Accountability allows autonomy. However, with the advent of "gatekeepers" and regulations from the insurance industry, some believe the autonomy so long characterizing health care is eroding (Swick, 2000).

ASHA's Ad Hoc Committee on Professional Autonomy defined autonomy as follows:

> An autonomous profession is one in which the practitioner has the qualifications, responsibility, and authority for the provision of services which fall within its scope of practice . . . Even the most entrenched professions are closely scrutinized and their practices repeatedly reviewed by bodies established by federal and state statutes, by accreditation agencies, by consumer groups, and by peers in the same profession. With the growing involvement of governmental agencies and corporations in underwriting the costs of human services, and with the growing trend for challenging professional competence through litiga-

tion, there is an ever-increasing abridgement of the independence of all professions. (ASHA, 1986, p. 53)

This may sound a bit contradictory, but Frattali (2001) clarifies in writing that

implied in the definition of professional autonomy, then, is the responsibility for formulating standards for preparation for practice, defining the scope and standards of practice, crafting codes of ethics, and developing both personal and institutional standards for the delivery of services to individuals with communication and related disorders. (p. 174)

Another component of accountability is being a lifelong learner, which, as stated earlier in this chapter, is a key element in professionalism. Swick (2000) points out that the majority of professions have as a foundation "intellectual work, a specialized body of knowledge, and expertise" (p. 613). These foundation blocks provide us with a "commonality" that enables us to agree, and sometimes disagree, with each other; it allows us to educate each other as we share our experiences and research; it enables us to maintain a state of excellence through programmatic reviews and standards.

Accountability allows autonomy. "Autonomy is a privilege granted by an external authority" (Swick, 2000, p. 613) and professionals who can demonstrate honest and sincere accountability will earn the privilege of being autonomous. However, professionals who view work as an entrepreneurial endeavor, as opposed to a collegial effort, will not be as respected as other professionals (Swick, 2000). Thus, as professionals, not only are we expected to be accountable to ourselves, but also to the profession as a whole. Whenever one of us is unprofessional, or unethical in our actions, we potentially have a negative reflection on our entire profession, which, in turn, could have a negative impact on our accountability and autonomy.

Accountability and autonomy are not the only factors that define a professional. Swick writes that health care professionals always will be faced with ambiguity and uncertainty, but a true mark of a professional is the ability to make independent decisions while handling the daunting conditions in which we sometimes find ourselves. These potential conflicts of interest may affect our decision, but a true professional will be able to weigh the impact of his or her choices, then make the decision that best meets the needs of the client.

Because its content seems appropriate in light of the prior information in this chapter, with the permission of Dr. Frederic W. Hafferty, I am reprinting a segment of an editorial response written in the *New England Journal of Medicine* (March 1, 2007).

> All sociocultural and occupational groups routinely normalize their life and work practices and settings. One consequence is that appreciable segments of a group's daily routines slip uncritically beneath any such "professionalism radar." Efforts to monitor the workplace for issues of professionalism should therefore be not only organized and proactive but also hypervigilant. Outsiders (those who are not part of the occupational group with its assumptions about the way things are and should be) thus need to be involved in the monitoring process. Patients are one such group. Others include new recruits, members of other (related and unrelated) occupational groups, and trained social observers such as anthropologists and sociologists. The ultimate goal is high quality patient care, and professionalism is too important a part of this praiseworthy effort to be left solely to insiders. (p. 966)

## Conflict of Interest Defined

Conflict of interest is defined by Resnick (1993) as "a dynamic tension between the private interests and the official responsibilities of a person in a position of trust" (p. 81). Examples of instances in which conflict can arise in our profession come from industry-supported research, commercial relationships between practitioners and product providers, working as an ENT office employee or partner, managing a hearing/speech/language center owned by an ENT physician, and working as a hearing aid dispenser as an outside contractor in the physician's office. These are examples of settings and transactions that require a balancing of one's professional ethics with one's business.

The Ethical Practices Board of the American Speech-Language-Hearing Association (ASHA) defines conflict of interest in the following way: "Situations where personal and/or financial considerations compromise judgment in any professional activity or where the situation may appear to provide the potential for professional judgment to be compromised." ASHA warns that it is critical for clinicians to maintain objectivity. Anything that brings into question the lack of objectivity should be avoided in all settings. ASHA goes further in writing four primary guidelines regarding the acceptance of gifts or benefits. Specifically, ASHA states that "speech-language pathologists and audiologists should not accept gifts or benefits unless it can be clearly demonstrated that such gifts or benefits

a. contribute to the welfare of persons served professionally
b. do not reasonably appear to bias professional judgment
c. enhance one's professional knowledge and skills
d. do not diminish the dignity or autonomy of the profession. (ASHA, 2004, p. 3)

Conflict of interest in the medical profession reached prominence as an issue in 1990 when the American Medical Association (AMA) scrutinized the pharmaceutical companies' relationship with physicians. The AMA paid particular attention to the physicians' prescribing patterns and their relationship to gifts from the pharmaceutical manufacturers. For example, pharmaceutical companies were offering all expense paid trips to physicians and their spouses. Others offered frequent flyer miles per prescription written, $100.00 for reading the literature on a toxic, non-FDA approved drug, and so forth. On the basis of this study, the AMA Council on Ethical and Judicial Affairs (1/1/91) said it is unethical to accept standardized vacations, cash gifts, cash for Continuing Education opportunities, and lavish meals and entertainment. Any gifts accepted by the health care professional should primarily benefit the patients and be of little value (less than $5.00), and should have minimal value and be related to work (notepads, pens). Money to reduce registration fees for continuing education opportunities can be accepted by the conference sponsor, but not by the physician. It is acceptable for a health care agency to sponsor scholarships, but the faculty must choose the student recipients. Finally, no gifts with strings attached can be accepted. In 1989, total pharmaceutical sales were $32.4 billion with at least $5 billion spent on marketing with averages out to $8000 per physician. Similar problems may arise with audiologists accepting gifts from hearing aid equipment manufacturers, and prescribers of augmentative/alternative communication devices accepting perks for recommending devices from a specified company (Resnick, 1993).

According to Swick, (2000, p. 613) there is an "expectation that a professional will subordinate self-interest" and this, too, can be considered a hallmark of a professional. With the increased "business-ization" of health care, many health care workers are sometimes thrown into a conflict between what the health system dictates and what the individual patients need. In adhering to the Code of Ethics for speech-language pathologists, the speech-language pathologist is charged with holding the welfare of patients paramount over all other potential conflicts of interest that the professional may face ("Individuals shall honor their responsibility to hold paramount the welfare of persons they serve professionally or participants in research and scholarly activities and shall treat animals involved in research in a human manner.") (ASHA, 2003).

Furthermore, and just as important, if not more than the profession's Code of Ethics, come the moral and ethical values that most health care professionals have that play a role in how we conduct ourselves personally and professionally.

Another area of potential conflict of interest lies in the "potential conflicts of interest in health care services and research" (Golper & Brown, 2004, p. 67). If a researcher is presenting his work, he needs to identify funding sources and/or vendors who have a financial investment in the research and could potentially influence the results. Likewise, if negotiations occur between a vendor and a facility as a result of research they funded, a conflict of interest would need to be reported to the facility.

**Task Block 1:** Brainstorm situations that a speech-language pathologist may encounter that could be construed by a consumer as a conflict of interest.

## Summary

Hannah Arendt states that authority's hallmark is "unquestioning recognition by those who are asked to obey; neither coercion nor persuasion is needed" (Arendt, 1969, p. 145). She goes on to cite Mommsen who makes the point that authority is less than a command and more than advice. Latham (1999) sums up the term "professional" by writing that these individuals make a "profession" that "is fundamentally a speaking-forth in public, before the world and before one's fellow professionals. It is a public commitment to obeying socially accepted standards both of morality and of competence in one's work . . . These are the acts of profession—the promises made by (health care professionals) to their patients and to their communities that they will use their expert authority wisely, and will not abuse it for the sake of money or power" (pp. 192–203).

# References

American Association of Medical Colleges. (1998). *Report I: A frame of reference for review and evaluation of medical school curriculum.* Washington, DC: Author.

American Speech-Language-Hearing Association. (1986). The autonomy of speech-language pathology and audiology (Report by the Ad Hoc Committee on Professional Autonomy). *Asha, 28,* 53–56.

American Speech-Language-Hearing Association. (2003). *Code of ethics.* Rockville, MD: Author.

American Speech-Language-Hearing Association. (2004). *Conflicts of Professional Interest* [Issues in Ethics]. Available from www.asha.org/policy

Arendt, H. (1969). On violence. In H. Arendt, *Crises of the republic* (p. 145). New York: Harcourt Brace Jovanovich.

Cruess, S. R., Johnston, S., & Cruess, R. L. (2004). "Profession": A working definition for medical educators. *Teaching and Learning in Medicine, 16,* 74–76.

Frattali, C. M. (2001). Professional autonomy and collaboration. In R. Lubinski & C. Frattali (Eds.), *Professional issues in speech-language pathology and audiology* (2nd ed.). San Diego, CA: Singular.

Golper, L. C., & Brown, J. E. (2004). *Business matters: A guide for speech-language pathologists.* Rockville, MD: American Speech-Language-Hearing Association.

Latham, S. R. (2002, November). Medical professionalism: A Parsonian view. *Mount Sinai Journal of Medicine, 69*(6), 363–369.

Pelligrino, E., & Thomasma, D. (1981). A philosophical reconstruction of medical morality. In E. Pellegrino & D. Thomasma (Eds.), *A philosophical basis of medical practice.* Oxford: Oxford University Press.

Resnick, D. M. (1993). *Professional ethics for audiologists and speech-language pathologists.* San Diego, CA: Singular.

Swick, H. M. (2000). Toward a normative definition of medical professionalism. *Academic Medicine, 75,* 612–616.

Wynia, M. K., Latham, S. R., Kao, A. C., Berg, J. W., & Emmanuel, L. (1999). Medical professionalism in society. *New England Journal of Medicine, 341,* 1612–1616.

# Chapter 16

# Conflict Resolution

*No man resolved to make the most of himself can spare time for personal contention. Still less can he afford to take all the consequences, including the vitiating of his temper, and the loss of self-control. Yield larger things to which you can show no more than equal right; and yield lesser ones, though clearly your own.*

Abraham Lincoln

## Introduction

In the workplace, it is almost inevitable that times of conflict between two or more employees will arise. Although conflict typically has a negative connotation, conflict often can lead to creative problem-solving. Rasberry and Lindsay (1994) write that, "conflict can add to a greater understanding and identification of problems. It can increase alternatives and involvement. Conflict stimulates interest and interaction. Hoffman, Harburg, and Maier observed that conflict encourages creative thinking, commitment, and quality decision-making" (p. 458). The purpose of this chapter is to discuss how to transform conflicts into opportunities.

## Setting the Stage for Dialogue

Cloke and Goldsmith (2000) stress the need to set the stage for dialogue as a critical component of conflict resolution. This can be accomplished by choosing a neutral site (go for a walk; eat lunch with your opponent) in which to engage in a conversation. In the conversation, one should be open and friendly instead of accusative and hostile. Honesty is a key factor; encourage your opponent to be honest in his or her assertions and responses and vow that you will also be honest in your assertions and responses.

When facing a conflict, many of us have a fight-or-flight response. If we engage in the "fight," there is a strong possibility that the levels of hostility and resentment will remain high, leading to a counterproductive environment in which to try to resolve the presenting conflict. Again referencing Cloke and Goldsmith (2000), successful conflict resolution requires that you clear your mind of everything you think you already know about the conflict, and listen empathetically to your opponent. Specifically, they recommend the following approaches and actions:

1. Learn from your conflicts by listening to them
2. Think of conflict as a request for communication
3. Use active, responsive, and empathetic listening
4. Understand others
5. Control your emotional responses
6. Don't take the conflict personally
7. "The largest part of your own anger often has nothing to do with the person to whom you are directing it, but everything to do with their actions and behaviors" (p. 15).

It also is important at the beginning of the resolution meeting that all individuals involved clearly state their emotional needs and self-interests, and listen carefully to those expressed by others. All participants should ask for what they want or need. You cannot "give up your anger and negotiate as equals" unless you do so. "Giving in to anger only encourages the conflict, cheapens the victory, and makes the other side look good, or permits them to dismiss your integrity and willingness to listen" (Cloke & Goldsmith, p. 15).

Look below the surface of what is being said to resolve the underlying reasons for the dispute. These reasons typically revolve around "communication breakdowns; poor performance; failure to follow policies and procedures; competition for scarce resources; misunderstandings about procedures, responsibilities, values, or goals; personality conflicts; and failure to cooperate" (Rasberry & Lindsay, 1994, p. 459). The issue being argued often is not the source of the conflict. "Issues that lie beneath the surface need to be brought into the open for conflicts to be resolved" (Cloke & Goldsmith, 2000, p. 15). Start with yourself and ask yourself what you can do to respond more appropriately and powerfully to your opponent's actions.

**Task Block 1:** Recall an experience you have had as a member of a group where there were conflicts among the members. How was the conflict resolved?

## Resolving Conflict

A key factor in successfully resolving a conflict is the ability to separate the person from the problem, the future from the past, and positions from interests. When the problem becomes an "it" instead of a "you," conflict transforms into opportunity. Debating can inhibit the process and make achieving a resolution much more difficult. Therefore, the participants should identify the interests of each individual, then begin dialogue to discuss these interests and determine why those interests are important. When individuals conflict over a position, there are very few possible resolutions; dealing with interests opens up multiple opportunities for resolution. Interests will enhance the choices you have, and assist you in looking toward the future (Cloke & Goldsmith, 2000). Cloke and Goldsmith remind us that we cannot change the past; the future is the sole component of conflict over which you have any control.

The next step is to brainstorm all potential solutions to your conflict, listing as many as possible, and ask the other person(s) to work with you to develop criteria to reach a resolution. Together, all involved persons can search for alternatives that will benefit all those who are affected by the decision/resolution. This is more likely to produce a compromise as opposed to a victory/defeat resolution that leaves half the persons involved with an unhappy and frustrating conclusion (Cloke & Goldsmith, 2000).

There are two types of strategies in conflict resolution: "outcome-directed strategies (who gets what) or goal-directed straregies (what would benefit both)" (Rasberry & Lindsay, 1994, p. 463). Rasberry and Lindsay cite the work of Filley who devised three forms of conflict strategies. The first is win/lose. In this scenario, individuals in the conflict seek to "make points" with those in charge, or to win an argument. Such individuals do not have the organization's goals at the forefront of the decision-making. The win/lose strategy often leads to deadlock and lack of resolution in the best interest of the organization. Filley (1977) provides four examples of win/lose situations. One is the dominance of power or authority in which things get done because an individual or group in a position of authority exerts this power through statements such as "I'm the boss and this is the way we are going to do this task." Another consequence of a win/lose strategy to conflict resolution is that not everyone will support the decision and may even go so far as to sabotage the implementation of the decision. A third approach is majority rules, which often involves taking a vote that results in a "winner" and a "loser." A fourth win/lose approach to conflict resolution is railroading, which usually involves coercion or applying pressure via undesirable consequences if the individual does not "go along with" our own point of view on the issue at hand.

Filley's second strategy is lose/lose which implies that there is no winner. However, it can also be thought of as compromising because each side of the conflict loses something it wanted.

The win/win strategy is the most desirable of the three, and it is one of two types: integrative and consensus. An integrative approach "focuses on a series of steps. It stresses goals and values and de-emphasizes solutions and win/lose tactics" (Rasberry & Lindsay, 1994, p. 466). Resolution by consensus focuses "on solving the problem rather than on the solution itself" (Rasberry & Lindsay, 1994, p. 465). When using consensus, the group proposes and analyzes several options to solving the issue at hand and eventually proposes a variety of solutions that could meet the needs of all involved individuals.

Successful resolution of conflicts is much more probable when the participants negotiate collaboratively rather than aggressively, and when they look for values, standards, or rules that will help resolve the dispute fairly, to everyone's mutual satisfaction (p. 16). When working collaboratively, participants are more likely to agree "on a set of shared values, standards, or mutually acceptable ground rules" (Cloke & Goldsmith, 2000, p. 16).

Use informal problem solving, mediation, and other conflict resolution techniques to overcome impasse, clarify areas of agreement, and reach closure. Let go of your judgments about your opponent(s) and focus instead on improving your own skills at handling their difficult behaviors. Then let go, forgive yourself and the other person, and move on with your life. "Your judgments about people are often distractions, ways of admitting you don't know how to respond skillfully to their behaviors" (Cloke & Goldsmith, 2000, p. 17). Rasberry and Lindsay (1994) note three techniques for resolving conflict: negotiation, mediation, and arbitration. In negotiation, it is possible that those in command may use covert or overt power plays in order to accomplish their goal. They also may bluff their way into dominance. In many ways, negotiation is a "bargaining process." Three types of negotiation include overt and covert negotiation, and bluffing. In overt negotiation, the negotiating group/individual makes promises, threats, or clues to communicate its stance. In covert negotiation, the negotiator tries to "subvert or contain the opponent" (p. 471) through the use of secretive maneuvers. Bluffing involves "creating a perception of power and its use" (p. 471). When using a bluff, the negotiator typically misrepresents the facts or prevaricates, and it is more effective in short-term negotiation than in long-term. Furthermore, it is easy to cross the line into unethical behaviors such as coercion and harassment when bluffing.

Rasberry and Lindsay propose the following steps to effective negotiation:

1. Do not confuse people with the problem. Keep them separate.
2. Avoid positional bargaining. Determine underlying interests, and then focus on them.
3. Do not select a solution while under pressure. This may limit its creativity and value. Consider as many possibilities as you can.
4. Agree on criteria or standards for measuring the effectiveness of the solution. Insist that objective standards be used. (p. 473)

In mediation, a third party who is neutral to the conflict acts as a "go-between" among the arguing factions. "Mediators must determine the problem, gather information necessary for its resolution, get and maintain involvement of the disputing parties, defuse emotions, analyze the complaint and determine alternatives" (Rasberry & Lindsay, 1994, p. 474). A mediator explains each side's perspective to the other side(s) and promotes efforts to achieve reconciliation between all parties involved.

An arbitrator is an appointed individual who, after hearing all sides of the conflict, is bestowed with the decision-making authority.

Typically, an arbitrator is called in when negotiation and mediation have failed. The arbitrator is selected by the involved parties and has legal authority to resolve the dispute. While a mediator tries to resolve the difference between the warring factions, an arbitrator makes the decision, which is then communicated to the conflicting parties (Rasberry & Lindsay, 1994).

The point is not to avoid conflict but rather to turn it into collaboration and an opportunity. Do not surrender just so the conflict will go away. This can lead to a buildup of resentment and frustration because it fits in with the "someone won and someone lost" attitude, which is counterproductive and does not lead to a satisfactory resolution. Instead, recognize the larger organizational and social issues that express themselves through conflict, and discover how your committed actions and acceptance of responsibility contribute to a more peaceful world (Cloke & Goldsmith, 2000).

Rasberry and Lindsay (1994) propose a six-step problem-solving model. The first step is to define the problem in terms of what the symptoms and effects are on all involved, and then to state the problem. The effects of the problem often result in conflict that will need to be managed through careful and decisive conflict resolution. The second step is to analyze the problem. In order to analyze the problem, it is necessary for each side (and/or the leader[s]) to gather the facts, to ascertain possible etiologies, then to set criteria to measure the extent of the problem. Third, possible solutions to the problem should be proposed. If the problem involves a difference of opinion between "sides," conflict arises. In this case, ideas to solve the problem should be generated. Each party involved should be willing to compromise (discussed elsewhere in this chapter) in order to reach a resolution in how the problem will be solved.

The fourth step is to select the solution. In this step, all possibilities for solving the problem are evaluated against the criteria to choose the best option. The plan is then implemented (step 5), with authority being delegated to various individuals or groups of individuals. Finally, the plan should be evaluated to see if there are any new problems, or if the plan needs to be revised in any manner. Rasberry and Lindsay point out that individuals or groups of individuals may be at varying stages of the problem-solving process at any one time, and that the steps are not necessarily sequential. Brainstorming often results in ideas that could be part of a stage not yet reached, or part of a stage already implemented. They write that "sharing perceptions, knowledge, and hypotheses helps to create understanding and support for the solution" (p. 427).

Cloke and Goldsmith (2000) stress the importance of searching for completion. "Summarizing what the other person said, asking them to feed back to you what they think you said, and making sure nothing is held back are useful strategies in allowing you to end the conversation and walk away feeling something has been transformed" (pp. 17–18).

## Facing Disagreement or Conflict

Conflict at home and/or work is inevitable. What defines our integrity is how we deal with the conflict. Goodwin (2006) proposes four steps to provide guidance in dealing with conflict and finding the best solution for all involved. The first step is, "Don't put the other person down" (p. 156). It is critical that the issue be the object of one's focus, not the person. It is easy to make a demeaning or condescending comment in the turmoil of an argument. However, "it is important to preserve the integrity and self-respect of all parties" (p. 156).

A second step is to "search for common ground" (Goodwin, 2006, p. 156). This necessitates that those in the midst of a conflict should try to see things from the other person's perspective" (p. 156). If the combatants can do this, they can hear what others have to say and find a foundation on which to build a solution.

Goodwin (2006) writes that the third step toward resolving a conflict is to "not expect behavioral changes" (p. 156). Conflict resolution needs to occur so that those involved can agree on what has to be done; they do not necessarily require a behavioral change.

Finally, Goodwin (2006) notes that one should not feel like he or she lost the argument just because he or she agrees to a compromise. "The goal is to find the best solution to improve productivity (reach agreed-upon goals), not to discover who might be right or wrong" (p. 156).

Indeed, compromise is often the best solution for all involved. Compromise is effected when each side of the conflict gives up and/or gains something. Through a problem-solving/decision-making approach such as compromise, a decision can be made with which each side is comfortable that the final conclusion is satisfactory, even though it may not represent everything each side wanted.

There are common phrases that reflect conflict as war versus conflict as opportunity, and conflict as a journey. Cloke and Goldsmith provide several examples of phrases that fit into the category of war, opportunity, or journey.

As war (p. 25)

"Your position is indefensible."

"We shot down that idea."

"We've got a battle on our hands."

"He dropped a bomb on me."

"I won."

As opportunity (p. 27)

"This difficulty presents us with a real challenge."

"Your feedback has given me some ways to improve."

"We now have a chance to make things better."

"What are all the possibilities for solving this problem?"

"Let's work together to find a solution."

As a journey (p. 29)

"Your idea points to a solution."

"This isn't getting us anywhere."

"Where do you want to go with that?"

"Let's do it together."

"I think we've arrived at an agreement."

"Let's search for common ground."

There are reasons we choose one strategy over another (Verbatim lists from pages 40-42). One strategy is to avoid or dodge the conflict. There are several reasons one would choose this strategy, even though it does not resolve the conflict. Specifically, Cloke and Goldsmith (2000) enumerate seven reasons for avoiding or dodging conflict:

1. You regard the issue as trivial.
2. You have no power over the issue and cannot change the results.
3. You believe the damage due to conflict outweighs its benefits.
4. You need to cool down, reduce tensions, or regain composure.
5. You need time to gather information and cannot make an immediate decision.
6. You can leave it to others who are in a position to resolve the conflict more effectively.
7. You regard the issue as tangential or symptomatic and prefer to wait to address the real problem.

### *Reasons for Accommodating or Giving in to the Conflict*

1. You realize you were wrong or want to show you can be reasonable.
2. You recognize that the issue is more important to others and want to establish good will.
3. You are outmatched or losing, and giving in will prevent additional damage.
4. You want harmony to be preserved or disruption avoided.
5. You see an opportunity to help a subordinate learn from a mistake.

### *Reasons for Aggression or Engaging in the Conflict*

1. You want to engage in quick, decisive action.
2. You have to deal with an emergency.
3. You are responsible for enforcing unpopular rules of discipline.
4. You see the issues as vital and you know you are right.
5. You need to protect yourself against people who take advantage of collaborative behavior.

### *Reasons for Compromise or Negotiating the Conflict*

1. Your goals are moderately important but can be satisfied by less than total agreement.
2. Your opponents have equal power and you are strongly committed to mutually exclusive goals.

3. You need to achieve a temporary settlement of complex issues.
4. You need a quick solution and the exact content does not matter as much as the speed with which it is reached.
5. Your efforts at either competition or collaboration have failed, and you need a backup.

*Reasons for Collaborating or Using Teamwork to Resolve the Conflict*

1. You believe it is possible to reach an integrative solution even though both sides find it hard to compromise.
2. Your objective is to learn.
3. You believe it is preferable to merge insights that come from different perspectives.
4. You need a long-range solution.
5. You want to gain commitment and increase motivation and productivity by using consensus decision-making.
6. You want to empower one or both participants.
7. You see it as a way to work through hard feelings and improve morale.
8. You want to model cooperative solutions for others.
9. You need to help people learn to work closely together.
10. You want to end the conflict rather than paper it over.
11. Your goals require a team effort.
12. You need creative solutions.
13. You've tried everything else without success. (Adapted from Thomas-Kilman Instrument by Cloke & Goldsmith, 2000).

A key to successful conflict resolution is to employ effective communication approaches for speaking with others. The following methods to encourage others to listen to you are suggested by Cloke and Goldsmith (2000, pp. 65–66).

1. *Before you speak, draw out the other person's ideas.* Start speaking by listening, so your ideas will be targeted and presented to your listener effectively. This does not mean watering down what you want to communicate, merely recognizing there are a multitude of ways you can say what you mean so the other person will be interested.
2. *Discover and manage your listener's expectations.* Make sure you do not base your comments on false expectations regarding

what the other person wants or is willing to do. Do not encourage others to have false expectations for you.

3. *Choose an appropriate form of speaking.* Decide what you want to communicate, and choose the form of communication that does what you want. If you want to make a declaration, make it an "I" statement rather than an accusation. Make sure your questions are genuine and not disguised statements. Be clear when you make a promise that you mean it.

4. *Speak respectfully, responsively, and emphatically.* Make sure you speak respectfully to the other person, *especially* when you disagree with them or disapprove of their behavior. Make sure you are responsive to the issues they have with you, and speak as you would want someone to speak to you.

5. *Put the listener at ease.* Speak informally, or in a way that relaxes the listener and encourages their trust in what you have to say.

6. *Demonstrate you have heard the other person's deeper needs and feelings.* Make reference as you speak to their issues and feelings, which may not be apparent at first glance. Demonstrate you are paying attention to what they have been telling you by summarizing their remarks without watering them down.

7. *State your interests rather than your positions.* Rather than repeating what you want, explain in a personal way why you want it.

8. *Anticipate objections and address them before they are raised.* Try to anticipate what the other person will say in response. Address those issues preventively before they do, as a way of demonstrating you understand their concerns.

9. *Acknowledge differences and restate issues positively.* Acknowledge your differences openly and state them neutrally, then restate the issues positively so they can be resolved. Afterward, test for understanding, agreement, and disagreement.

10. *Clarify and emphasize your agreements.* Do not lose sight of what you actually agree on. Start by thanking the other person for agreeing to discuss their issues openly with you. If they have done so, emphasize earlier points of agreement, whatever they are. There have to be some things you agree on, even if it is only your agreement to talk directly with each other rather than ignore the problem or take it to someone in authority.

11. *Focus on developing solutions.* Address problems that can be solved rather than attempting to assign blame for unsatisfactory conditions.

12. *Ask questions of the listener.* Asking questions is usually more powerful than speaking. At the end of your comments, turn the conversation over to the listener by requesting a response to what you said, or ask questions that could result in changing your mind.

13. *Compliment the other person for listening.* Give positive reinforcement to the other person for listening and indicate your willingness to listen to them with an open mind (Phrases for Miscommunication from Cloke and Goldsmith, pp. 67–68).

The following items represent phrases for miscommunication that create a combative atmosphere as opposed to an atmosphere in which those in the conflict can work together toward a resolution (Cloke & Goldsmith, 2000, pp. 67–68).

1. *Ordering:* "You must _____," "You have to _____," "You will _____"

2. *Threatening:* "If you don't _____," "You'd better or else _____," "You'll pay a big price _____"

3. *Preaching:* "It's only right that you should _____," "You ought to _____," "It's your duty _____"

4. *Interfering:* "What you should do is _____," "Here's how it should go _____," "It would be best if you _____"

5. *Judging:* "You are argumentative (lazy, stubborn, dictatorial . . .)" "I know all about your problems." "You'll never change."

6. *Blaming:* "It's all your fault." "You are the problem here."

7. *Accusing:* "You lied to me." "You started this mess." "You won't listen."

8. *Categorizing:* "You always _____," "Every time this happens you do the same thing _____," "You never _____"

8. *Excusing:* "It's not so bad." "It wasn't your problem." "You'll feel better."

9. *Personalizing:* "You are mean." "This is your personality." "You are the problem here."

10. *Assuming:* "If you really respected me, you would _____," "I know exactly why this happened."

11. *Diagnosing:* "You're just trying to get attention." "Your personal history is what caused this to happen." "What you need is _____"

12. *Prying:* "When? How? What? Where? Who?" "What are you hiding?"

13. *Labeling:* "You're being unrealistic (emotional, angry, hysterical . . . )" "This is typical of you _____"

14. *Manipulating:* "Don't you think you should _____," "To really help you should _____"

15. *Denying:* "You did not _____," "I am completely blameless _____"

16. *Double binding:* "I want you to do it my way, but do it however you want."

17. *Distracting:* "That's nothing, listen to what happened to me _____"

**Effectively listening** (pp. 70-78). On the other hand, Cloke and Goldsmith (2000) propose phrases that can facilitate the resolution of conflicts:

*Let go of your own ideas, roles, and agendas, and try to understand what the other person is saying* (p. 70)

1. Prepare yourself to listen

2. "Am I open for learning and poised to understand what he is saying, or thinking about what I am going to say in response?" (p. 71)

3. Search for the other person's meaning, especially if they disagree with you
   a. Listen for intended message, not just spoken message.
   b. What do they really want? What are their real intentions?
   c. What is going on beneath the surface?" (p. 71).

4. Respond respectfully and nondefensively, acknowledging and addressing the other person's concerns first (p. 71).
   a. "Respond by addressing the speaker's point of view, rather than immediately countering with your own and ignoring most of what they said" (p. 71).

    b. "Thank you for your information. I appreciate hearing your point of view" (p. 71).

    c. Don't replace their ideas with yours.

5. Active and Responsive Listening Techniques
    a. Encouraging (p. 72)
        (1) "Please tell me more"
        (2) "I would like to know your reactions"
        (3) "I hear what you are saying"
    b. Clarifying (p. 72)
        (1) Focus on facts rather than feelings
        (2) "When did this happen?"
        (3) "Who else was involved?"
        (4) "What did it mean to you?"

*Acknowledging* (p. 73)

1. Name the feelings the speaker is expressing
2. "I can see you feel angry about that"
3. "I can appreciate now why you might feel that way"

*Normalizing* (p. 73)

1. "Communicate to the speaker that it is natural and normal to have those feelings"
2. "I think I might feel the way you do if that had happened to me"

*Empathizing* (p. 73)
1. Put yourself in other's shoes to better understand their feelings and perceptions
2. "I can understand why you feel strongly about this subject because I experienced something similar in my own life"
3. "I can appreciate why you might feel that way"
4. "I understand"
5. Don't say "I understand exactly how you feel"

*Soliciting* (pp. 73–74)

1. "I would like your advice about how we could resolve this"
2. "What do you think should be done?"
3. "Tell me more about what you want"
4. "What would you like to see happen?"

*Mirroring* (p. 74)

"Reflects back the emotions, affect, demeanor, body language, tone of voice, metaphors, even breathing patterns used by the speaker to encourage the speaker to feel they have a companion in their thoughts and emotions rather than a dispassionate observer."

*Agreeing* (p. 74)

1. "What I like about what you just said is _____"
2. "I really agree with you about that. What I think we disagree about is _____"

*Supplementing* (p. 74)

1. "Let me build on that and see if I am on the same track you are"
2. "Let me support what you are saying with another point"
3. "Not only that, _____"

*Inviting Elaboration* (pp. 74–75)

1. Ask open questions
2. "Why?"
3. "What would you like to see happen?"
4. "Why is that important to you?"
5. "I'd like to ask you a question about that."
6. "How would you _____?"
7. "Help me understand why you _____."

*Reframing* (p. 75)

1. "Preserving the content of a communication but altering its form so it can be heard and possibly result in a solution"
2. Helps identify the reasons for disagreement
3. Reframe your statements as statements
4. "I feel [whatever] when you [do whatever], because [reason]"

*Responding* (p. 75)

1. "Listening respectfully means responding to what is said, not using listening techniques to manipulate the speaker."
2. "If I understand you correctly, you see the problem this way [summary]. Here's how I see it."

3. "Would you like to know how I see it?"
4. Make your point clear, but do not be defensive or angry in your responses

## Summarizing (p. 75)

1. "Let me see if I understand what you just said _____ [summary]. Is that correct?"
2. Provides speaker "opportunity to confirm, correct, or change your understanding of the communication"

## Validating (p. 76)

1. "Recognize the speaker's contribution and thank them for communicating with you"
2. "I appreciate your willingness to raise these issues with me"
3. "I learned a great deal from what you said"
4. "I know it took a lot for you to be as open as you were and I want to acknowledge you for taking that risk."
5. "I appreciate your willingness to talk with me about this."
6. "I didn't know you felt that way before."

## Empathetic Listening

1. "Become one with the speaker and discover *their* truth within you" (p. 77)
2. Deeper than active listening
3. "It requires you, the listener, to focus on awareness not just on the words the other person is using but on what they may be thinking or feeling. It means asking yourself what it would feel like to be in their shoes and what would cause you to make that statement or communicate that way yourself" (p. 77)

## "Listen for: (p. 77)

| | |
|---|---|
| Subjective experiences | Interpretations |
| Roles | Modes of perception |
| Intentions | Emotions and feelings |
| Interests and positions | Wishes and desires |
| Dreams and visions | Family patterns |

| | |
|---|---|
| Fears | Insults and stereotypes |
| Humiliations | Self-esteem |
| Defensiveness | Resistance |
| Denial | Prejudices |
| Metaphors | Apologies |
| Universality | Uniqueness |
| Cries for help | Expressions of guilt |
| Openings to dialogue | Desire for forgiveness |
| Requests for acknowledgment | Need for support" |

## Summary

Conflict is not always negative; in fact, it can be a healthy component of problem-solving and decision-making. Rasberry and Lindsay (1994) write that, "if participants accept this principle and apply problem-solving skills, then greater commitment, more creative alternatives, and sounder decisions will more than likely result" (p. 594).

## References

Cloke, K., & Goldsmith, J. (2000). *Resolving conflicts at work: A complete guide for everyone on the job.* San Francisco: Jossey-Bass. Reprinted with permission of John Wiley & Sons.

Goodwin, C. (2006). *Supervisors's survival kit* (10th ed.). Upper Saddle River, NJ: Pearson Prentice-Hall.

Filley, A. C. (1977). Conflict resolution: The ethic of the good loser. In R. C. Huseman, C. M. Logue, & D. Freshley, (Eds.), *Readings in interprersonal and organizational communication* (3rd ed.). Boston: Holbrook Press.

Phillips, D. T. (1992). *Lincoln on leadership.* New York: Warner Books.

Rasberry, R, W., & Lindsay, L. L. (1994). *Effective managerial communication* (2nd ed.). Belmont, CA: Wadsworth.

# Chapter 17

# Stress and Burnout: How to Recognize It and How to Tackle It

*What lies behind us and what lies before us are tiny matters compared to what lies within us."*

Oliver Wendell Holmes

## Introduction

Stress, which is defined in *Webster's New Universal Unabridged Dictionary* (1996) as "a specific response of the body to a stimulus, as fear or pain, that disturbs or interferes with the normal physiological equilibrium of an organism" (p. 1882). Everyone experiences stress at some time or another, but the response of the body to stress varies from individual to individual. Some have psychological responses and some have physiologic responses, but no matter how one defines stress or responds to stress, it is known to be detrimental to efficiency and effectiveness in all settings, and can lead to strained relationships with our family, our friends, and our coworkers.

## Personal Issues and Problems Due To Stress

Butler and Hope (1995) wrote a chapter on stress in their book, *Managing Your Mind*, in which they identified internal and external sources of stress. Internal stress includes our wants, feelings, and attitudes. External sources of stress develop in our homes, our work places, and other settings in which we sometimes find ourselves. External sources of stress may include any pressure you are under and/or any burdens you may be carrying. Internal stress sometimes occurs as a reaction to our external sources of stress.

Stress can produce social/pragmatic and health problems. Social/ pragmatic issues could be exhibited as having trouble concentrating on a communication exchange, being short-tempered with family and/or friends, being "on edge," and possibly withdrawing from social settings or other settings that require interaction with others. Butler and Hope write that health problems such as bowel problems, headaches, and heart attacks are known side effects of stress, with heart attacks being most prevalent. In addition, existing illnesses such as asthma, skin rashes, arthritis, and epilepsy can get worse if an individual has these medical problems.

Cloke and Goldsmith (2000) cite the work of Howard Friedman in which he analyzed existing research that looked at the effect that people's state of mind has on their physical health. They write that as a result of his research, Friedman found "that being chronically pessimistic, irritated, cynical, depressed, and anxious doubles the risk of contracting a major disease. There is a link between the emotional centers of the brain, the immune system, and the cardiovascular system" (p. 80).

The interaction of brain chemicals and stress hormones that occurs in reaction to negative emotions also can affect our physical health affecting our susceptibility to cancer, high blood pressure, and high cholesterol, making us more prone to develop any of a variety of illnesses.

Butler and Hope (1995) identify four steps to decide if you are getting stressed:

1. Learn to recognize your own signs of stress
2. Weigh the size of the load
3. Think about recent changes in your life
4. Think about recent changes in yourself.

With regard to learning to recognize your personal signs of stress, they list the following questions one should ask him or herself to see if any specific factor plays a role in creating stress:

1. What does it feel like when you are stressed?
2. How does it show?
3. What thoughts run through your mind?
4. What do you do?
5. How does it affect others?
6. How do their reactions affect you?

The first question, "What does it feel like when you are stressed?" guides us in identifying the social and/or physical reactions we have to stress. Stress may show up in the workplace, and at home, as reduced efficiency that is visible to others as evidenced by dragging our feet and avoiding making decisions. "What thoughts run through your mind?" is a question that can help us realize "who," "what," or "when" factors that may be at the root of our stress by deciphering how our thought processes govern how we react to any of these situations— a location, an event, or a person. The reactions we have to stress can be divided into four groups: feelings, thoughts, behaviors, and sensations. These reactions are listed in Table 17–1.

**Table 17–1.** Changes That May Be Signs of Stress

**Feelings**

Irritability; you become short-tempered, or easily flare up

Anxiety or feelings of panic

Fear (e.g., of being out of control)

Feeling worried (e.g., about your health, or anything else)

Feeling miserable or tearful

Apathy or agitation

Lowered self-esteem

**Thoughts**

Forgetting things; making mistakes

Finding it hard to concentrate

Becoming indecisive

Getting muddled or confused

*continues*

**Table 17–1.** *continued*

**Thoughts** *continued*

Procrastinating

Being unable to think far ahead

Worrying or ruminating rather than solving problems

Becoming rigid and inflexible, in an effort to keep control

Predicting the worse

**Behaviors**

Getting worse at managing your time

Getting worse at organizing yourself, and others

Rushing hither and thither

Finding it hard to delegate

Working longer and longer hours

Bringing work home; working on weekends

Avoiding tackling problems, or doing things you dislike

Cutting down on the things you do for pleasure

Losing touch with your friends

Blaming others for the problem

Taking it out on others ("kicking the cat")

Finding there's no time to enjoy yourself

Needing a drink; turning to drugs

Needing tranquilizers or sleeping tablets

**Sensations**

Aches and pains, especially headaches or stomachaches

Tension (e.g., in your neck and shoulders)

Frequent minor ailments

Disrupted sleep patterns

Appetite for food increased or decreased

Appetite for sex increased or decreased

Ulcers

Flare up of stress-related illness, such as asthma or psoriasis

*Source:* From *Managing Your Mind* by G. Butler and T. Hope, p. 211. Copyright Oxford University Press, 1995. Reprinted with permission.

Weighing the size of the load is a second way to identify if you are under stress. One way to do this is to write down the stresses you face, both small and large. This helps you focus in on what situations, people, expectations of others, and/or settings tend to provoke a state of stress. Also, stressors can be prioritized by making a note whether the stressor was major, moderate, or minimal. Butler and Hope (1999) also suggest not comparing your reactions to stresses to those of others or your previous reactions to that stressor. For example, they advise against making statements such as, "Everyone else copes with this" or "I should be able to cope; I could last year." Another trap is to discount or minimize your load because this "only adds internal stress to the external load and puts you under more pressure" (Butler & Hope, 1999, p. 210).

A third strategy to help identify your own stressors is to think about recent changes in your life. Major and minor changes are part of everyday life. However, change saps one's energy, which means that there is not as much energy to deal with daily issues until one has adjusted to the change, being able to integrate the impacts of change into one's mode of functioning (Butler & Hope, 1999). Stressors identified in the two previous steps will consume one's energy, compounding the effects on one's mental, physical, psychological, social, and vocational capabilities.

The final step in the identification process it is to think about recent changes in one's self. Table 17-2 lists some of these personal changes.

### *Dealing with Stress*

The two most common and/or fundamental means of dealing with stress are tightening up and turning away, or relaxing and turning toward the source of the stress.

> When we withdraw from our emotions, we end up learning little or nothing about what gave rise to then, or how to experience them fully, or how to respond to them skillfully, or how to recognize what lies underneath them. When we relax, let go of our fear of expressing emotions, and engage them, we release ourselves from their grip and increase our clarity, creativity, opportunities for learning, and chances for resolution, transformation, and healing. (Cloke & Goldsmith, 2000, p. 81)

**Table 17–2.** Examples of Stressful Events*

---

**Major Changes**

Changing jobs

Getting married, separated, or divorced

Business readjustments

Pregnancy

Moving house

Leaving school, or changing schools

Outstanding achievement

Getting or losing a mortgage

Retirement

**Losses**

A friend or relative dies

People you are close to move away

Children leaving home

Stopping work

Giving up work to have children

**Disruptions in routine**

Vacations, Christmas, bank holidays

Someone new in the home (e.g., a friend or a new baby)

Stopping smoking or drinking

Dieting

No opportunity for exercise

**Trouble and strife**

Arguments, especially with a partner

Brushes with the law

Illness

Injury

Financial problems.

---

*Note: These are not in order of severity. That depends on you.

Source: From *Managing Your Mind* by G. Butler and T. Hope, p. 213. Copyright Oxford University Press, 1995. Reprinted with permission.

It is not healthy to deny, avoid, or suppress our emotions, and these actions can result in our not formulating a resolution to the problems, and possibly lead to conflicts within ourselves and with others. Rather, rationally and constructively handling the emotions that occur as a result of stress can lead to clarification of the reason for the stress, and enable one to more fully cope with the stressing issues or events (Cloke & Goldsmith, 2000).

Butler and Hope (1995) issued two notes of caution when experiencing stress. One is to "make sure that the solutions you use will be helpful in the long term as well as in the short term" (p. 212). Sometimes, one puts a Band-aid on a stressor by making a quick fix of the issue, rather than thinking through the impact that this quick response may have make in the long term. This, in turn, can eventually produce stress because the stressor grew in proportion to the ultimate impact from the effectiveness of the short-term solution.

The second cautionary statement is not to consume caffeine. It is well documented in the medical literature that caffeine can cause tension headaches. Because stress also can result in headaches, the consumption of caffeine in stressful situations can lead to worsening physiological responses such as headaches.

When you cannot get stress under control, try these four steps (Butler & Hope, 1995)

1. **Take stock of the situation.** It is a good idea to take a moment to stop and think through the situations that are creating stress. When stress increases, there is a need to have breathing space to evaluate the situation. This will help one put things in perspective, and minimize the consumption of energy that the stressor is producing.
2. **Start with the end in mind.** When one has clarified his or her priorities, he or she is better able to make decisions that will lead to a less stressful, balanced life. Clarifying priorities based on the desired end-results will also serve as a guide to making small decisions. As discussed earlier, some small decisions become big ones when they are not acted on immediately, and if the short-term solution potentially does not match the desired end-point, more stress will occur. It is also important to put priorities into practice. If a person claims that spending time with his or her family is the number one priority but spends 50 to 70 hours a week working,

he or she may feel increased stress because he or she is not putting his priority list into effect.

Define basics and priorities, and then think about dealing with the effects of stress through a variety of actions. One action is to write things down. Stress can adversely affect one's ability to concentrate and to remember people, events, and necessary tasks. Butler and Hope (1995) also suggest scheduling planning time every day. "Stress makes planning and decisions difficult" (p. 215). Some people find that planning time first thing in the morning helps to clarify the day, whereas others may find it helpful to have planning time in the evening or at the end of the work day to line things up and create the action priorities for the next day.

Give yourself breaks for meals, snacks, and exercise because stress can cause fatigue. It is important, Butler and Hope point out, to stop and engage in these activities before reaching a point of exhaustion. It is also helpful to eat a healthy diet. For example, instead of heading for the soda pop machine, head to the local juice bar. It is also important to minimize stress because stress can lower one's resistance to illness and can slow down one's speed of recovery.

Because stress can make one feel pressure more acutely, it is important to minimize and/or take the urgency out of the daily routine and life in general. Some techniques for this are found in the time-management chapter. Keeping a time diary may help to minimize urgency that results in stress while simultaneously increasing efficiency.

3. **Reduce the "outside" and "inside" loads** (Butler and Hope list these separately, but I have combined them for sake of discussion). Again referencing Butler and Hope, our attitudes ("inside") toward how we prioritize, and how we deal with our stressors ("outside"). Remember, stress can be cumulative, so deal with the small problems before they become stressors. It may be necessary to change one's attitudes to minimize the loads that lead to stress. Attitudes can make the difference between increasing or decreasing pressure. In Table 17–3, attitudes that result in increased and decreased pressure are compared.

4. **Lay the right foundation.** "Feeling stressed is a danger signal: a sign that you are reaching the limits of your resources. Stress is bad for your physical health as well as a cause of increasing inefficiency and worsening relationships" (Butler & Hope, 1995, p. 217).

**Table 17–3.** Stressing Statements Versus Stress-Relieving Statements

| *Putting the Pressure On* | *Taking the Pressure Off* |
|---|---|
| I have to get this done. | I will do as much as I can during the allotted time. |
| I shouldn't ask for help. | Everyone ask for help sometimes. I would happily help someone else. |
| This is really important. | In five years this won't matter at all. When I'm on my deathbed, I won't be saying, "I wish I'd spent more time in the office." |
| I must do things well. | I can only do my best. |
| Others cope far better than I. | Everyone is susceptible to stress. I am not alone in this. |
| There's nothing I can do. | Try solving the small problems first. |
| I'll crack up completely. | I need a break, so I'll take a break. |
| I can't let anyone see how I feel. | There's nothing to lose by talking to someone about my feelings. |

*Source:* From *Managing Your Mind* by G. Butler and T. Hope, p. 216. Copyright Oxford University Press, 1995. Reprinted with permission.

As stated earlier, it is important to eat regular, healthy snacks and meals. Exercise is a wonderful stress reducer and does not have to be overly time consuming. Taking a 15-minute walk during a midafternoon break is helpful in dealing with stress. Rest, recreation, and relationships are also important stress managers. Because stress can self-perpetuate in a vicious cycle, one needs "rest, to renew your energy; recreation, to provide you with pleasure and fulfillment; and relationships, as a source of support and perspective" (p. 217).

## What Stressors Are Identified in Different Work Settings?

The author conducted a small survey of speech-language pathologists working in a variety of settings, asking four questions related to stress and burnout:

1. Rate your job's stress level with 5 being the highest and 0 being "no stress."
2. What is the number one stressor in your job?
3. What is your best "stress relief" strategy.
4. Have you ever experienced burnout and, if so, how did you overcome it?

The results of this survey are in Table 17–4. Across settings, it is apparent that paperwork and time demands are the most prevalent stressors. One of the responses from individuals in private practices came from the owner of the practice that may have affected her answers with regard to money being the worst stressor. With regard to how stressful we find our jobs, from setting to setting we were fairly consistent in considering our jobs to be moderately stressful overall. This is not to say we do not have days where our stress level is higher than average or lower than average, but when averaged out, most of us conclude that a middle level of stress is the most prevalent. It speaks well of us in terms of our relationship with our patients/students that several individuals indicated that one of their best stress relievers involved interacting with those individuals who enlist our help in remediating their communication deficits.

**Table 17–4.** Stressors and Burnout Expressed by SLPs in a Variety of Settings

| *HOSPITAL-AFFILIATED OUTPATIENT CLINIC* |
| --- |
| **#1 stressor** |
| 1. management |
| 2. time to complete work/paperwork and staying up on many areas |
| 3. productivity (2) |

**Table 17–4.** *continued*

4. budget

5. paperwork

**Best stress relief strategy**

1. talking/conversing with peers

2. don't know

3. commiserating over coffee with my office mate (2)

4. biking

5. taking a lunch break or taking a walk at lunch

**Experienced burnout/how overcame it**

1. yes; changed settings from inpatient to outpatient

2. yes; took a break from work

3. yes; took a vacation

4. yes; I took a long (3-week) vacation

5. no

6. yes; I found new therapy materials to work with.

---

*HOSPITAL ACUTE*

---

**#1 stressor**

1. Not having time to do paperwork, phone calls, and therapy planning built into my day's schedule

2. productivity ratings (the facility focusing on money and not the patient. I have not conformed to this and must stand up to those stressors as a result.

3. time to complete work/paperwork and staying up on many areas

4. complicated cases

**Best stress-relief strategy**

1. going home and leaving all the work at work; go to be with family

2. focus on the patient and gain satisfaction from knowing that I am giving them my all

3. NR

4. walking outside and taking deep breaths

*continues*

**Table 17–4.** *continued*

**Experienced burnout/how overcame it**

1. yes/left the job and moved to another (have worked in 3 places but had burnout only once)
2. yes/through prayer and changing my personal focus to the patients and no the "politics" of the job
3. yes/took a break
4. yes, a vacation

**UNIVERSITY CLINIC**

**#1 stressor**

1. managing/maintaining a client census and clinical experiences to insure student training and competency attainment
2. not enough time to complete work at work and feeling pressure to work at home
3. changes in procedures/protocols/schedule
4. dealing with marginal students (doesn't happen often)
5. NR
6. Inefficiency (things that should be carried out easily and quickly become burdensome)
7. lack of respect and appreciation from students and my immediate supervisor
8. the unexpected time demands that occur
9. Too much to do and not enough time
10. too many responsibilities and too little time
11. not enough time
12. time pressure; scheduling clients simultaneously in an hour; not bad with experienced clinicians but a "killer" with rookies!
13. budget and staff limitations
14. timelines

**Best stress-relief strategy**

1. preplanning/projecting developing procedures to deal with problems
2. running/exercising
3. humor with colleagues
4. talking to coworkers

**Table 17–4.** *continued*

5. walking, reading, working in the garden, "daily glass of wine"
6. jazzercise right after work, which means leaving work on time (the hours I was hired for)
7. venting to friends; time with my dogs
8. exercise—walk around the buildings—leave for lunch (usually eat in)
9. finding humor whenever I can. Laughing with coworkers and students
10. still searching for it, but am trying to leave anything associated with work at the office and not think about it once I leave for home
11. exercise/yoga; not bringing work home
12. listening to music in my office; taking nothing home
13. 10-minute break in a room with no people in it
14. chocolate

**Experienced burnout/how overcame it**

1. no/loved public school and university settings
2. yes/took a sick day
3. yes/time off and consulting with the director to change things
4. yes/finding a new project to work on
5. yes in previous job/left after 17 years
6. yes/recalling client successes and focusing more on one preferred aspect of the job
7. yes/looked for a new job
8. yes/took a leave for 2 years and maintained regular hours when I returned
9. yes/I took a semester off
10. NR
11. not often/ I have good variety in my job
12. maybe a bit. Worked through it; tried learning new ways to do the same stuff
13. yes/switched settings
14. yes/attending conference in new area and implementing new knowledge

*continues*

**Table 17–4.** *continued*

| **SKILLED NURSING FACILITY** |
|---|

**#1 stressor**

developing continuity of care with dietary/nursing to meet patient needs

**Best stress-relief strategy**

go out for lunch/take a break/time away

**Experienced burnout/how overcame it**

yes/time off

| **ELEMENTARY SCHOOLS** |
|---|

**#1 stressor**

1. meeting needs of challenging students; dealing with teachers who are against/resistant to inclusive practices
2. paperwork
3. not having enough time to make documentation and analyze progress
4. NR

**Best stress-relief strategy**

1. talking and laughing with colleagues
2. therapy—direct contact with students
3. taking time for prayer and meditation and walking
4. I do not have one.

**Experienced burnout/how overcame it**

1. yes; cried a lot, then "regrouped" and looked for possible solutions
2. yes; changed jobs
3. yes; started a new project for the children and got very involved in my state association
4. yes; I overcame it by realizing that I made a difference in the lives of the children I work with.

| **PRIVATE PRACTICE** |
|---|

**#1 stressor**

1. finances: reimbursement and #2 staff retention and consistency (owner of own private practice)

**Table 17–4.** *continued*

2. time management—completing therapy activities, discussing therapy/evaluation with caregivers, and writing therapy notes within allotted time frame

**Best stress-relief strategy**

1. leave the building; going out to lunch is rare but great!
2. try to allow a few minutes between therapy sessions so that I am not rushed when speaking to caregivers, write down a brief summary of therapy activities and activities to complete at home to give to the caregiver

**Experienced burnout/how overcame it**

1. yes; change focus of therapy with new continuing education experience to try new techniques
2. yes; a few days of vacation works wonders for me. It is also helpful to discuss specific problems with coworkers

---

*COMMUNITY CLINIC*

---

**#1 stressor**

1. money—generating billable hours, finding/writing grants, paying expenses, etc.
2. managing the parents dealing with the stress related to raising a child with hearing loss, and coordinating therapy with the parent in the room
3. management

**Best stress-relief strategy**

1. focus on patient care (my passion) and 'me' time at home; being able to cross an item off my "to do" list
2. leaving work
3. working out

**Experienced burnout/how overcame it**

1. yes/what would I gain if I were in a different place or job? Asking myself this question helps me realize every age/season has its compensation
2. yes/working on overcoming it right now!
3. keeping a gratitude journal

## Burnout

Lubinski, Golper, and Frattali (2007, p. 5279) cite Maslach (1982) in defining burnout as "a syndrome of emotional exhaustion, depersonalization, and reduced personal accomplishment that can occur among individuals who do 'people work' of some type." Burnout among health care and education professionals can be the result of the complicated and persistent needs of our patients/students, our own personal stresses (including paperwork and lack of sufficient time to complete all duties) at home and/or in the workplace. Table 17–5, developed by Lubinski, Golper, and Frattali lists several sources of burnout.

In a survey by the author of fellow professionals in a variety of settings, the respondents were asked to report whether or not they had ever experienced burnout, and how they handled it. The results are shown in Table 17–6.

**Table 17–5.** Sources of Burnout

**Client Factors**
- Overly demanding clients and/or families
- Complicated, serious problems of clients and/or families
- Lack of client/family responsiveness
- Lack of client/family appreciation

**Professional Situation Factors**
- Size of caseload
- Lack of autonomy
- Little opportunity for self-actualization
- Low pay; few salary increases
- Job insecurity
- Little opportunity for continuing education
- Tedium
- Excessive paperwork and inadequate time to complete it
- Inadequate working conditions and/or resources
- Discrimination: sexism, ageism, racism
- Inadequate supervision

**Table 17–5.** *continued*

- Unclear criteria for professional evaluation
- Evaluation based on negative factors only
- Lack of coworker support
- Bullying behavior by coworkers
- Interdisciplinary conflict or competition
- Unprofessional attitudes on part of supervisor or coworkers
- Lack of positive reinforcement from supervisor
- Rigid or unrealistic institutional policies

**Personal Factors**

- Unrealistic expectations; perfectionism; need for control and to "do it all"
- Inability to say "no"
- Inability to delegate work to others
- Lack of confidence
- Need for approval from others
- Hostility
- Impatience
- Personal and/or family health problems
- Family pressures
- Competing demands of job and family

*Source: Professional Issues in Speech-Language Pathology and Audiology* by R. Lubinski, L. A. C. Golper, and C. Frattali, p. 530. Copyright 2007 by Thomson Delmar Learning. Reprinted with permission.

**Table 17–6.** Techniques for Handling Burnout

**Clinicians in Hospital-Affiliated Outpatient Clinics**

Changed settings from inpatient to outpatient

Took a break from work/vacation

Found new therapy materials to work with

**Clinicians in Acute-Care Hospitals**

Left the job and moved to another (have worked in 3 places but had burnout only once)

*continues*

**Table 17–6.** *continued*

**Clinicians in Acute-Care Hospitals** *continued*

Through prayer

Changing my personal focus to the patients and not the "politics" of the job.

Left the job

**Clinicians in University Clinics**

Took a sick day

Consulting with the director to change things

Finding a new project to work on

Recalling client successes

Focusing more on one preferred aspect of the job

Looked for a new job

Quit working overtime

Worked through it

Attending conference in new area and implementing the new knowledge

**Clinicians in Skilled Nursing Facilities**

Took time off

**Clinicians in Elementary Schools**

Cried a lot

Regrouped and looked for possible solutions

Changed jobs

Started a new project for the children

Got very involved in my state association

**Clinicians in Private Practice**

Change focus of therapy with new continuing education experience to try new techniques

Discuss specific problems with co-workers

Time off/take a vacation

**Clinicians in Community Clinics**

Considered what I would gain if I were in a different place or job

Realizing that every age/season has its compensation

Kept a gratitude journal

Cloke and Goldsmith (2000) write the following about stress and burnout: "It can produce quite uncharacteristic changes in someone's ability to function, leading to poor physical health, stomach ulcers, irritability, increased use of alcohol of caffeine, and eventually to 'burnout'" (p. 387).

Citing Cherniss (1980), Lubinski, Golper, and Frattali (2007) discuss the three stages of the process of burnout. In stage 1, there is an "imbalance between the demands and resources to deal with job stress" (p. 531). In instances such as this, the external demands from work/home/family/social aspects of one's life outweigh the internal resources and strategies to cope with the stressors. As a result, stage 2 occurs, which is signified by changes in one's feelings and health, with symptoms such as fatigue, tension, anxiety, and physiologic exhaustion. The individual is likely to exhibit signs of illness and weakened ability to fight off illness. In stage three, the individual may invoke "defensive coping" strategies such as "emotional detachment withdrawal, cynicism, and rigidity. Table 17–7 lists the signs and effects of burnout in terms of professional effects, psychological effects, physiologic effects, and effects on significant others.

**Table 17–7.** Signs and Effects of Burnout

**Professional Effects**
- Detachment/depersonalization
- Sense of inadequacy
- Irritation with clients
- Diminished listening skills
- Decreased work output
- Deteriorating work performance
- Leave work earlier than usual/increased absenteeism
- Negative impact on finances of individual or agency

**Psychological Effects**
- Sadness
- Anger
- Frustration
- Loss of satisfaction or accomplishment
- Overly self-critical

*continues*

**Table 17–7.** *continued*

**Psychological Effects** *continued*
- Cynical and negative
- Tension
- Anxiety
- Depression
- Forgetfulness
- Feelings of helplessness
- Suspiciousness
- More risk taking
- Paranoia
- Suicide

**Physiologic Effects**
- Feeling of exhaustion and chronic fatigue
- Reduced autoimmune response
- Increased susceptibility to illness and infection
- Rapid heart rate
- Hormonal abnormalities
- Shortness of breath
- Poor eating habits
- Addiction to controlled substances or alcohol
- Frequent headaches
- Insomnia
- Gastrointestinal disorders
- Dermatologic disorders (e.g., hives, eczema, acne)
- Back and neck disorders
- Hypertension
- Heart attack
- Stroke

**Effects on Significant Others**
- Marital conflict
- Family discord
- Loss of intimacy
- Estrangement from others

*Source:* From "Stress, Conflict, and Coping in the Workplace," by R. Lubinski. In R. Lubinski, L. A. C. Golper, and C. Frattali (Eds.), *Professional Issues in Speech-Language Pathology and Audiology* (p. 532). Copyright 2007 by Thomson Delmar Learning. Reprinted with permission.

## Closing Remarks

The focus of this chapter has been on the stress associated with being a professional in a work setting as well as at home. As health care professionals, we should be alert to the fact that the caregivers of many of our patients experience this type of stress at home, too. Knowing the signs of stress can alert a speech-language pathologist to the need to assist out patients' and/or their caregivers in finding effective outlets to reduce their stress, and to provide maximum support to these wonderful individuals.

## References

Butler, G., & Hope, T. (1995). *Managing your mind: The mental fitness guide.* New York: Oxford University Press.

Cloke, K., & Goldsmith, J. (2000). *Resolving conflicts at work.* San Francisco: Jossey-Bass.

Lubinski, R., Golper, L. A. C., & Frattali, C. (2007). *Professional issues in speech-language pathology and audiology.* Clifton Park, NY: Thomson Delmar Learning.

# Index